THE REPRODUCTION REVOLUTION
New Ways of Making Babies

STUDIES IN BIOETHICS
General Editor *Peter Singer*

Studies in Bioethics is a series aimed at introducing more rigorous argument into the discussion of ethical issues in medicine and the biological sciences.

THE REPRODUCTION REVOLUTION

New Ways of Making Babies

PETER SINGER and
DEANE WELLS

Oxford New York Melbourne
OXFORD UNIVERSITY PRESS
1984

Oxford University Press, Walton Street, Oxford OX2 6DP

London Glasgow New York Toronto
Delhi Bombay Calcutta Madras Karachi
Kuala Lumpur Singapore Hong Kong Tokyo
Nairobi Dar es Salaam Cape Town
Melbourne Auckland

and associated companies in
Beirut Berlin Ibadan Mexico City Nicosia

Oxford is a trade mark of Oxford University Press

Published in the United States
by Oxford University Press, New York

ISBN 0 19 217736 2
ISBN 0 19 286044 5 (pbk)

Set by Hope Services
Printed in Great Britain by
Richard Clay (The Chaucer Press) Ltd
Bungay, Suffolk

PREFACE: THE NEW ERA

On 25 July 1978, in Kershaw's Cottage Hospital in Oldham, Lancashire, Louise Brown was born. With her was born a new era in making babies. Until then, every human being had begun her or his existence deep inside a female body. There, unseen by human eyes and protected from any kind of outside interference, egg and sperm had fused and the fertilised egg had begun the process of dividing and growing that leads, if all goes well, to the birth of a baby nine months later.

Louise Brown was different. Not different in her appearance, which was just like any other healthy new-born girl. Nor was this normal appearance in any way deceptive. Beneath the surface, too, there was nothing different about her. Louise Brown was a normal baby and is now a normal child. It is her history that is different.

Lesley and John Brown had been wanting children for several years, but Lesley Brown was infertile. Her ovaries produced eggs, but the eggs could not pass down her Fallopian tubes to be fertilized. Surgery to remove the blockage proved unsuccessful. Then she was referred to Dr Patrick Steptoe, an Oldham gynaecologist, who, together with the Cambridge biologist Dr Robert Edwards, was working on a novel method of overcoming infertility.

What Edwards and Steptoe did was to remove an egg from one of Lesley Brown's ovaries, place it in a glass dish, and then fertilize it with her husband's sperm. This is easy to say, but much harder to do: we shall say more about the method shortly. For the Browns, the significance of the technique was that it enabled them to have a longed-for child; but Edwards and Steptoe accomplished something much more momentous than that. For the first time, a human being had developed from an egg that was fertilized outside the female body. Thus Edwards and Steptoe opened a door on a host of new possibilities in the field of human reproduction. With these possibilities come great hopes, but also great fears. Suddenly we are faced with an array of new ethical issues: the permissibility not just of the method used to create Louise Brown, but also of the freezing of human embryos, the use of surrogate mothers, the use of embryos for 'spare parts', and, of course, cloning.

Until the birth of Louise Brown these issues were the kind of thing that might interest science-fiction writers, but for the ordinary public they were too remote to be worth serious thought. Now they have come upon us with a rush, and there is a need to make complex decisions that could well determine not just *how* our grandchildren come into existence, but *who* they are—their genetic identity.

These issues are too important to be left to the scientists and doctors who are creating the breakthroughs. There must be public discussion involving the entire community. Then some tough decisions will have to be made. We have written this book as a contribution to this process. We begin with a prologue, suggestive of the possibilities of the new era in human reproduction. The book itself consists of two parts. In the first we look at the basic process which made possible the existence of Louise Brown and the many other children who have since been conceived by the same technique. We describe the procedure, as seen through the eyes of a couple taking part in it, and we consider in some detail the ethical debate stirred up by it. Included in this section, because they are already in practice, are the issues of egg donation, embryo donation, and embryo freezing. In the second part of the book we look ahead—but perhaps not very far ahead—to ways of making babies that have not yet been tried, but are either already technically possible, or else likely to become technically possible in the near future: true surrogate motherhood (in which the surrogate is not the genetic mother of the foetus she carries); ectogenesis, or development outside the womb; cloning; sex selection; and genetic engineering.

We have been fortunate in receiving assistance from many people. The work has been carried out at the Monash University

Centre for Human Bioethics. It was begun under a grant from the Myer Foundation which enabled Alan Rassaby to work on several aspects of *in vitro* fertilization; we have drawn particularly on his work on surrogate motherhood. A subsequent grant from the National Health and Medical Research Council of Australia made it possible for Deane Wells to join the project. Others at the Centre have made valuable contributions, especially Helga Kuhse with the section of Chapter 3 on the moral status of the embryo, and Margaret Brumby with information on opinion polls. (In this latter instance we must also thank the Roy Morgan Research Centre for making their data available to us.) Most importantly, without John Swan and Bill Walters the Centre for Human Bioethics itself would not have existed and so those interested in the issue could not have come together in the fruitful way they have. To Bill Walters we owe additional thanks, for it was he who first drew the attention of one of us (P.S.) to the ethical issues raised by the attempts—as they then were—of Carl Wood's team to achieve *in vitro* fertilization.

We must also thank several researchers who have provided us with information on their work: Carl Wood, Alan Trounson, and John Leeton at the Queen Victoria Medical Centre, and Ian Johnston and Alex Lopata at the Royal Women's Hospital. In England, Robert Edwards and Patrick Steptoe made time available for discussions, and sent us papers. We had useful meetings with Mary Warnock and Peter Quilliam. Clifford Grobstein, from the Center for Science, Technology, and Public Affairs at the University of California, San Diego, also assisted us in gathering data.

Patsy Littlejohn worked with us on a questionnaire for patients on the Queen Victoria Medical Centre IVF programme. In this connection we must thank Carl Wood and the Medical Centre for allowing us to administer the questionnaire, Jillian Wood for seeing that the patients got it, and the patients who completed it.

For permission to describe their personal experiences with IVF we are most grateful to Jan and Len Brennan and to Isabel and Toby Bainbridge. We also thank Faye Bland for allowing us to use the details of the birth of her son Kim, at the beginning of Chapter 5, and Margaret Tighe for agreeing to be interviewed on the stance taken by Right to Life Australia.

Margaret Brumby and Anne McLaren each made valuable comments on the typescript.

Finally, and very gratefully, we thank Lynette Anderson, who typed some of the book on a playfully-inclined word processor, and Jean Archer, who typed most of it in her usual splendid way.

The views expressed in this book are, of course, our own. In particular, they are not necessarily those of the Centre for Human Bioethics, the Myer Foundation, or the National Health and Medical Research Council.

December 1983   P.S.
                                                       D.W.

CONTENTS

Note on currencies

Sums of money are given in their native currencies.
The abbreviation used for US dollars is $ and that
for Australian dollars $A. Currency conversion
rates at the time of going to press were:

$$£1 = \$1.46$$
$$£1 = \$A1.6$$
$$\$1 = £0.69$$
$$\$1 = \$A1.09$$
$$\$A1 = £0.63$$
$$\$A1 = \$0.91$$

PROLOGUE: A TWENTY-FIRST-CENTURY DINNER PARTY

It was one of those social events that caused the hosts a little anxiety beforehand. John and Jacqueline had been lucky enough to get a transfer to the same school. Their fellow teachers, they had found, were easy to get on with—first names all round and so on. The teaching year had begun, and was in full swing with no hitches. Their colleagues were no longer strangers, but were still largely an unopened book to the two new members of staff. So Jacqueline and John had taken the step of inviting several of them to dinner. They were both looking forward to the event, but as they hurried around, arranging seating and checking the automatic food dispensers, they were hoping that they had invited compatible dinner guests. Class and religion were not particularly divisive issues in the mid-twenty-first century, but the widespread high technology of the time made available such a variety of private life-styles, that people who got on well at one level (such as the work-place) often found each other bewildering in another environment. John and Jacqueline knew nothing of the private lives of their guests. That was the souce of their anxiety.

The doorbell rang. That in itself was significant. It was fashionable for most homes to give visitors the option of ringing a bell or selecting a tune, just by pressing a button. Whoever was at the door was not giving anything away.

'Guess who it is!' Jacqueline challenged her husband, as she went to the door.

'That's probably Christine', he guessed correctly.

Christine was welcomed in. She was tall and athletic-looking and always appeared composed. John and Jacqueline thought of her as being about as assertive as one can be without being overbearing.

Almost immediately the door played the opening bars of 'Thus Spake Zarathustra'.

'That's Raymond', they all said at once.

So it was. More precisely, it was Raymond and his wife Rachel. Raymond was the school's Principal, and he and Rachel ran their lives on a pattern that was more familiar in the twentieth century, although a substantial minority still did similarly. Raymond was what was known colloquially as a patriarch. He was a dominant male, and head of his family. His wife had not worked since their marriage (if indeed she ever had) and she had borne him four children. Raymond made decisions for them both, even such decisions as which button to press at the front door. He had chosen to advertise his arrival with a stirring fanfare.

The guests were seated and the drinks trolley came around. Raymond keyed in a request for a whisky for himself, and a pink gin for Rachel. Soon more music was coming from the portals. This time it was a carefree little tune from a popular song.

'That will be David', said Raymond, who knew his history master well. But when John got to the door he found David's wife, Angela, with her finger on the button. The newcomers seemed to be similar in much more than their musical tastes. They walked to their seats with a similar fluid stride, and both spoke in a soft but arresting tone of voice. When drinks came around again, each selected a newly fashionable cocktail.

The arrival of David and Angela completed the guest list, and John immediately dialled up the meal. He had programmed the main course, and Jacqueline had programmed the soup and the dessert. Their recipes were a great success, and after the meal the room was filled with the relaxed hum of conversation. There was a lot of shop talk, but nobody was left out. Rachel and Angela were entirely at home talking about the school. Rachel's main interest in life outside the home centred on Raymond's career, and Angela, who was a scientist, was as interested in the activities of her talented historian husband as he was in hers. But the conversation drifted to other things as well, as people followed their own interests with others who shared them.

Then the whole room was galvanized into unity by a chance event. Jacqueline had been talking to Rachel about the four children she and Raymond (but mainly she) were bringing up, when Jacqueline mentioned that she and John were going to have a baby. It just happened that there was a lull in the conversation at that moment, and everybody heard her news. There were congratulations all round, but none so enthusiastic as those of the headmaster and his wife.

'Well done, well done!' said Raymond, and then after a pause, 'I suppose we'll be losing you for a while then, Jacqueline?'

'Not just yet though', she said, 'I'll be with you until the final term and then I'd like time off until the baby is born.'

'And after that Jacqueline will come back for the first term. I would like to take the first term off to look after the baby', John said.

Raymond raised his eyebrows. The request was common, and he would not be refusing it, but deep down he felt that it was Jacqueline who should be taking first term off next year.

'But Jacqueline', said Rachel, 'don't you want to be with your baby after it's born?'

'Of course she does', John interposed, 'but there is no reason for her to lose touch completely with what's happening at school, especially when I'm so keen to spend time with the baby. We've wanted a child for six years, and we're going to share it when it comes.'

'Did you say six years?' Rachel asked in astonishment. 'We had our first less than a year after we were married. Why did it take so . . .', and then she stopped, realizing why. Nearly all infertile couples availed themselves of the public *in vitro* fertilization facilities, and there was always a long waiting-list. Even so, six years was a long time, as everyone in the room realized.

John knew that nobody would be rude enough to ask for further explanation, but he also knew that everyone would be interested. 'There was a further complication. We thought for a while we were going to use artificial insemination as well as *in vitro* fertilization, but we didn't have to in the end. The baby will be genetically Jacqueline's and mine. With a little help from the doctors I managed to deliver the necessary goods', he joked, and his guests all laughed.

Raymond however had laughed out of politeness. Initially he had been delighted that his new staff members were having a baby. But then he had discovered that they were availing themselves of this 'new-fangled' paternity leave. He thought of it as new, though it had been customary for decades. When he had discovered that they were in fact having a 'test-tube baby'—as Raymond still thought of it—he had no moral objection to that. Why should 'infertile' couples be discriminated against? And he knew that with the technique John and Jacqueline were using, the baby didn't really grow in a test-tube—it was only the fertilization that took place outside the body. All the same, he felt he had more in common with people who did it all the old way, just like he and Rachel had. He looked at his wife and knew she was thinking the same.

'I'm afraid I'm going to have to ask you for paternity leave too', David said to Raymond.

'Good heavens, when is *your* baby due?' said Raymond, too surprised to offer the customary congratulations.

'Not baby—babies', said David, 'It's quadruplets.'

All eyes turned to Angela, but there was no evidence of it.

'The year after next', said Angela, answering Raymond's question.

'So you are going to have quads the year after next . . .', said Jacqueline slowly. The implication was left hanging, questioningly; and when David and Angela nodded, everyone present drew the obvious conclusion. The young couple had had their genetic material frozen, to be stored for a year or so, when it would be nurtured by ectogenesis. It had to be ectogenesis. No one *chose* to be quadruply pregnant. The practice of ectogenesis was comparatively recent, but no longer rare. Like David and Angela, modern-minded couples were avoiding pregnancy by arranging for their future family to spend its first nine months in a laboratory.

After a silence it was Jacqueline who spoke first. 'Do you really mean it?' she asked Angela. 'Wouldn't you rather feel close to your baby the way one does in pregnancy?'

'I can't carry them all can I?' Angela replied gently. 'At least one of them would probably die.' She and David knew they would have to go through this sort of event a number of times, and they were not going to allow themselves to become ruffled.

'That's true', said Rachel, 'but you could have them one at a time.'

'We want them all at once', said Angela. 'There are lots of advantages for children who have twin brothers and sisters. And now that sex selection is also available, we will have a perfectly planned family.'

'Those advantages far outweigh any advantages a child has by being carried around by its mother for nine months', David confidently added.

'But that's a rather male-oriented view, don't you think David?' said Raymond. 'There's a certain bonding that goes on between the mother and child in those nine months. Surely a mother couldn't love her child as much without it?'

'Do you think that you love your children inadequately?' David asked Raymond.

The question was aggressive, but Raymond knew he had provoked the aggression, and simply answered in the negative.

'But you didn't carry your children around in your body for nine months, did you? So why do you imagine that Angela won't love our children enough?'

'Oh, nobody said she wouldn't love them enough', Jacqueline put in hastily. 'We just thought that perhaps she might love them even more than that if she was pregnant with them.'

'And what precisely is the advantage to children of being loved more than enough?' David asked. 'Enough is enough. Anyway, what you say doesn't make sense. There's no scale for measuring love. Either parents love their children enough to do what is in their best interests or they don't. We are going to.'

'Fair enough', said John. 'But don't you think it might be in their interests to be born after a pregnancy? There must be something in the bonding theory.'

'You sound like that twentieth-century novel where all the babies were mass-produced in anonymous hatcheries,' said Angela. 'If there is anything in bonding, it cuts two ways. We will be going to the laboratory to see them every day. David will actually feel closer to them than he would otherwise. In a pregnancy a woman can't see her baby but she can feel it. A man can't do either. David will actually see our children developing day by day.'

'Apart from all that', said David, 'it's in the children's interests to have a happy and fulfilled mother, just as it's in my interests to have a happy and fulfilled wife. Angela now has a brilliant scientific career ahead of her, and it wouldn't help if she was estranged from it for ten years having four babies successively. This way we can each take a year off, one after the other, and give the children our full attention in their formative years, without disrupting our careers.'

The other two couples were silenced, but not convinced. They still knew how they felt. Raymond was feeling rather more favourably disposed towards Jacqueline and John now. Perhaps they weren't quite doing it the old way, but they were close enough really. John's insistence on taking paternity leave was a bit soft line, Raymond thought, but perhaps the *in vitro* bit didn't matter. What was a medically necessary hospital conception compared to what these other two renegades were doing?

At this point Jacqueline turned to Christine, who had been sitting back all the while with a look of amusement that bordered on the supercilious. Christine was single, and Jacqueline thought it would be safe to make a joke around the fact so as to deflect the conversation to something more harmonious.

'Well, I suppose you don't have any surprises for us on this score do you Chris?' she asked.

'Actually, yes', she said, with a wicked look. 'I'm pregnant'.

'What?' several people exclaimed.

'Who's the father?' asked Raymond—a more personal question than he would normally have asked. Tonight, obviously, was not going to be a normal evening.

'There isn't a father', said Christine.

'You mean you don't know who the father is!?' Rachel was unable to control herself.

'You're impugning my modesty, or my discretion or something', said Christine. 'I mean, precisely, that there isn't a father.'

'You mean you are giving birth to your own clone?' said Angela slowly, with an unreadable smile.

'Exactly'.

Cloning had been possible for a few years, but was hardly ever practised. Any woman could do it, provided she didn't want a male child. She would herself supply the necessary egg, and the egg could be fertilized with material taken from any cell of her body. Her child would then have exactly her physical constitution, and would literally have no father. It was now the standard way of producing dairy cattle, of course, and one heard that women did it occasionally: but actually knowing someone who was doing it reduced all the diners to a state of shock.

'Why on earth are you doing it?' asked John, forgetting politeness and his special duties as host both at once.

'Because I want to have a baby', said Christine, deliberately forcing those she had just shocked to spell out their outrage.

'But how can you be so egotistical as to have yourself cloned?' asked Jacqueline.

'You and John have just gone to a lot of trouble to reproduce your genetic codes. The only difference between your egotism and mine is that yours is mutual between the two of you.'

'But what about your baby?' urged Rachel. 'Wouldn't it be better with a father?'

'Unless you're insulting my genetic structure', said Christine acidly, 'you are suggesting that children of single parent families fare worse than children of dual parent families. The experience of the last hundred years provides ample evidence that that isn't true, at least where poverty isn't a factor.'

They had all heard of the studies done on this issue, and knew that her claim was debatable, but Christine taught athletics, literature, and sociology, and her experience in the last field would guarantee that she would win the argument on the day. So nobody pursued it.

'What if, just for the sake of argument, of course', asked Angela impulsively, 'someone was to insult your genetic structure?' Her tone was so beguiling that Christine took no offence.

'I had it checked out beforehand of course', Christine said. 'Although I am never sick, and I'm physically very strong and can expect to live a long life, I have some recessive genes which carry serious hereditary disorders. One way I can guarantee that they don't become dominant in my daughter is by duplicating myself entirely, rather than chancing pot luck with sexual reproduction.'

'I suppose your daughter won't have much to complain about', said David, looking her up and down with exaggerated provocativeness.

'But it's so *unnatural*', said Rachel in an almost pleading voice.

'So are chocolate biscuits', said Christine, and coolly helped herself to another.

There was a long silence. Jacqueline began to talk about the new designs of flowering plants in the latest gardening magazine. The topic was hastily picked up by Rachel, and the conversation moved on to other subjects. By the time they all got up to go their separate ways, only the most acute observer would have noticed the slight awkwardness in their friendly partings.

*

As she drifted into sleep that night, Rachel echoed her husband's thoughts.

'I really don't like what those people are doing, you know. Don't you think the world would be a better place if people just let nature take its course?'

'Of course it would, darling', Raymond replied, as he checked the remote scanners to see his children sleeping peacefully at the other end of the house, checked the functioning of the computers which controlled the temperature and negative-ion generators, and flicked the switches on the bedside console to start the children's hypnopaedic in-sleep teaching programmes.

*

'Funny lot of new colleagues we've got', John said to Jacqueline, as they reflected on the fact that their dinner party had turned into exactly the event they had envisaged in their worst fears.

'I can't understand them at all', replied Jacqueline. 'I just can't see why they won't just let nature take its course.'

Then she drifted off to sleep, thinking about how nature, with admittedly a little initial impetus from science, was taking its course in her own body.

*

David and Angela hardly paused to look at their meticulously planned and tidy home before retiring to their bedroom. David called out to his wife as he dried himself in the shower in the *en suite*.

'Darling, you know it's still true that breast-feeding is best for babies. I've got a form from the hospital for the treatment so you can feed them all.'

Angela appeared at the door in her negligee.

'But darling', she said with mock reproachfulness, 'you can't possibly want me to breast-feed four of them. Think what it might do to my figure. Anyway let's not think about it now. Come to bed instead.'

*

Christine was at that moment lying in bed looking at her own baby photos. 'She's going to be a beautiful baby', she was thinking. Suddenly the phone rang. She felt a sudden jolt. She knew who it was, or at least she hoped she did. She was going to have to tell him what she had done, and that might be the end of them. Of course she could always let him think that . . . but then that wouldn't really be fair. She looked at the phone, back at the baby photos, then back at the phone, as if torn between two competing worlds. Then she picked up the phone.

PART I
The Present Scene

1 FERTILIZATION OUTSIDE THE BODY

Five years on

In vitro fertilization—literally, fertilization 'in glass'—is no longer an experiment. Six months after the birth of Louise Brown came Alistair Montgomery, the first IVF boy. Then another eighteen months went by before Professor Carl Wood's team at the Queen Victoria Medical Centre in Melbourne, Australia, successfully used *in vitro* fertilization to enable Mrs Linda Reed to have a daughter, Candice. For a time the success rate of the Melbourne team surpassed that of the English originators of the process. As the number of babies produced rose into double figures, the media fanfare that had greeted each birth declined, flaring again only for new developments, like the first IVF triplets, or the first pregnancy from a frozen embryo.

Now, five years after the birth of Louise Brown, *in vitro* fertilization is being used to treat infertile couples in medical centres in Britain, Australia, the United States, Germany, Denmark, France, Sweden, Austria, Italy, Singapore, and Israel. New centres are opening all the time, so this list will need constant updating. Changing even more rapidly is the tally of babies produced. It took two and a half years to reach double figures, but only another year to pass the hundred mark. It will grow even faster as the more recently established centres develop their expertise. *In vitro* fertilization has become an accepted treatment for some forms of infertility.

This success is, of course, the result of much more than five years work. The new treatment for infertility was made possible by the coming together of advances in two entirely separate fields of modern science: reproductive biology, and fibre optics. These two fields were united in the working relationship of Robert Edwards and Patrick Steptoe.

Edwards is the biologist. For his Ph.D. at Edinburgh University, he artificially inseminated mice with specially modified sperm, and observed the fertilization and early growth of the resulting mouse embryos. Then in 1960, a married couple who were close friends of his became concerned about their inability to have a child. One common cause of infertility, Edwards knew, is blocked or diseased Fallopian tubes. These tubes are the means by which a woman's eggs are carried down to the womb. If they are not functioning the woman will still be producing eggs, but they will have nowhere to go, and she will never become pregnant through sexual intercourse. But what if, Edwards wondered, the egg could be taken from the ovary where it is produced, fertilized in the laboratory with the husband's sperm, and then transferred to the womb? Could this be a method of overcoming childlessness for people like his friends?

This thought led to a long period of research, both with mice and with human eggs obtained from women who needed to have pieces of their ovary removed for medical reasons. For fertilization to take place, however, the eggs would have to be removed at just the right time, when they were properly ripe; this made it difficult for Edwards to obtain an adequate supply from operations conducted for a different purpose. Nor could he expect volunteers to have their ovaries cut up in order to provide him with eggs for his experiments.

Not until 1967 did Edwards find the path toward a solution to this problem. Browsing in a Cambridge library, he noticed a journal article by a gynaecologist called Patrick Steptoe. It was about something called 'laparoscopy'. This was then a novel way of examining the inside of a patient's abdomen without having to cut it open. The method was named after the instrument it used, a laparoscope. The laparoscope was a kind of thin telescope with its own light. It could be inserted in the abdomen through a small cut, and the doctor could then look through it. Early laparoscopes were only of limited use, however, because the lamp rapidly overheated. Then in 1964 a German instrument maker developed a laparoscope which used the recently invented system of fibre optics. Using hundreds of very fine glass fibres, it had been found that intense light could be conducted down the fibres, and even around corners. The fibre-optics laparoscope had no electrical connections and did not overheat.

Edwards and Steptoe teamed up in 1968, with the specific aim of helping infertile women to conceive by fertilizing their eggs outside the body and implanting them in the womb. Within a year they found the right culture fluid, in which the egg would continue to ripen for a few hours. They introduced the sperm, and fertilization occurred. Their results were published in the scientific journal *Nature*, in 1969, and soon newspaper headlines announced that human life had been begun in a test-tube. Ethical controversy began at the same time, with the experiments being condemned by the Archbishop of Liverpool, but receiving the support of the well-known social reformer, Baroness Summerskill.

After studying the growth of embryos in the culture, and assuring themselves that they grew normally, Edwards and Steptoe attempted to transfer them to patients. It took four years of fiddling with hormones before the first pregnancy occurred— and then this turned out to be an ectopic pregnancy; that is, the foetus was not growing in the womb but rather in what remained of the patient's Fallopian tube. In this situation, the foetus has no room to grow and it can burst the wall of the tube, threatening an internal bleeding which could be fatal for the mother. The pregnancy had to be terminated.

Further work produced a second pregnancy, but it spontaneously aborted in the first few weeks. It was not until December 1977 that tests confirmed the successful transfer of an embryo to a patient named Lesley Brown.

Meanwhile, in Melbourne, Carl Wood had been working on *in vitro* fertilization since 1970. Previously he had attempted to develop an artificial tube for women with diseased Fallopian tubes. The artificial tube, however, could not replicate all the functions of the natural tube, and so it did not work. At a conference of the Australian Society of Reproductive Biology, held in Melbourne in 1970, a paper was presented on the artificial tube, and an animal reproductive biologist suggested that as an alternative one might try techniques already in use in farm animals on quite a large scale. To produce more offspring from very valuable pedigree sheep and cattle, scientists working in the livestock industry had been using hormones to get the females to produce a large number of eggs. They had then artificially inseminated the animals, flushed the embryos out of the womb—for there were too many to survive—and then transferred them to the wombs of less valuable animals, who acted as 'surrogate mothers' for lambs or calves that were not genetically related to them. The animal biologist was suggesting that if the egg could be fertilized in the laboratory, the technique of transferring it back to the womb could be a way of getting around the problem of the blocked Fallopian tubes. (No one was, at that stage, suggesting the use of selective breeding or surrogate mothers for humans—although in view of the origins of the procedure, these were always possibilities, once IVF succeeded in humans.)

Wood thought the idea interesting enough to take a look at what was being done with sheep in Australia, and this in turn convinced him that the technique could hold the answer to the infertility problems of some women. He had also heard that Edwards and Steptoe were working on the same method in England.

A Melbourne team began work in 1971, and eggs were collected but attempts to fertilize them failed. By 1973 fertilization had taken place, and two patients were thought to have had an early pregnancy, but the pregnancies did not establish themselves. Further attempts were made until 1978, but none succeeded. Nevertheless when news of the success of Edwards and Steptoe reached Melbourne, the team had seven years' experience to draw on. It was therefore able to advance more rapidly than other overseas groups, and was the first to repeat the success of the Edwards/Steptoe team.

What's in a name?

Before we describe the techniques now being so widely used, a word about terminology. Babies produced by *in vitro* fertilization are often referred to as 'test-tube babies', a term with obvious appeal to those who compose newspaper headlines. The closest the procedure comes to putting babies in test tubes, however, is when an egg is put together with sperm in a glass container and, after fertilization takes place, kept there for two or three days. At this stage the embryo is not, by any stretch of the imagination, a baby. It consists of two, four, eight, or at most sixteen cells, all apparently alike. It is impossible to tell which cells will eventually form the head, or the limbs, or the placenta. In so far as the term 'test-tube baby' conjures up a picture of something recognizably akin to an infant, growing in a glass tube, the term is misleading (It would be better reserved for the future prospect of ectogenesis, or complete development outside the womb.)

'*In vitro*' is Latin for 'in glass', so '*in vitro* fertilization' simply means that the fertilization takes place in glass. Of course it would make no difference to the significance of the procedure if it could be done with equal success in plastic or wood or metal; but the term '*in vitro*' has come to be used, in a variety of scientific contexts, to make the contrast with something that happens '*in vivo*', that is, in a living organism. An alternative label, used by the American biologist Clifford Grobstein, is 'external human fertilization'. This has the advantage of summing up, in plain English rather than in Latin, exactly what is distinctive about the procedure; but Grobstein seems to have made his sensible suggestion too late. '*In vitro* fertilization', often shortened to 'IVF' is the term that has stuck, and is the term we shall use.

How is it done?

Rather than describe *in vitro* fertilization in the abstract manner of a scientific article, let us follow the experiences of one of the couples who have had a child by IVF. Many couples who have used IVF wished to retain their privacy; but Jan and Len Brennan have been happy to tell their story fully and frankly. We retell it here, not because they are a typical IVF couple—every couple is different in some way—but because it does reveal something of the nature of the treatment.

Jan and Len Brennan live in a Melbourne suburb. They were married when she was twenty-four and he was forty-one. It was her first marriage, but his second. They did not expect the marriage to result in children. When Jan was nineteen, she had gone to her doctor complaining of internal pain. The doctor said they were 'ovulation pains' and prescribed aspirin. It was not until the pain had persisted for four weeks that she was referred to a gynaecologist, who discovered a serious infection in both

Fallopian tubes. For a time her life was in danger; to save it, she underwent an operation in which her Fallopian tubes were removed. She survived, but was told that she would never have children of her own.

At nineteen, the thought of infertility was depressing; but it was only after her marriage to Len that Jan began to feel the full impact of her condition. As one female friend after another excitedly announced that she was pregnant, Jan felt an increasing emptiness and sadness at missing out on what they were experiencing. She also worried that Len would come to see their relationship as incomplete because it was childless. Jan and Len would have happily adopted a child, but a shortage of children for adoption has led Australian adoption agencies to exclude any couple in which one partner is over thirty-five. Even for couples under the cut-off age, there is a long waiting-list. For the Brennans there was no chance at all.

Early in 1978 Jan and Len asked their doctor to send them to a specialist, just to see if anything could be done. They were referred to Professor John Leeton, who, together with Professor Carl Wood, works in the Monash University Department of Obstetrics and Gynaecology. At this stage, however, Leeton could offer little hope. He merely suggested that they keep in touch, in case some new treatment turned up.

Something did turn up: Louise Brown. For the first time the Brennans began to hope. In March 1979 they received a letter from Leeton inviting them to receive treatment from a new IVF team then beginning work at the Queen Victoria Medical Centre. They accepted without hesitation, elated at having the chance of a child at last.

After preliminary interviews and tests, Jan's first attempt at IVF was in June 1979. There was a problem with the timing of her monthly cycle, and nothing could be done. Two months later she went again. This time she was given an anaesthetic and taken to the operating theatre. There John Leeton made three small cuts in her abdomen, below her navel. Into the first he inserted a laparoscope. Through the second cut Leeton put a hollow needle, just one millimetre in diametre, and through the third, forceps. Looking through the laparoscope, Leeton used the forceps to find the ovary and manoeuvre it into position so as to be able to get at the egg, ripening in a follicle on the surface of the ovary. He punctured the follicle with the hollow needle, which was connected to a vacuum pump. Fluid flowed up the needle, and an assistant filled test tubes with it. The tubes were rushed to an adjacent laboratory where Dr Alan Trounson, the senior reproductive biologist with the Monash team, examined them under the microscope. He found an egg.

The egg was kept in a suitable fluid for about six hours, to allow it to continue to mature fully—it was, after all, taken from the ovary before the natural process of development had released it. During this period, Len provided the semen, through masturbation. This was done in a private room, together with Jan.

The next stage is fertilization. The semen, with its hundreds of thousands of sperm, was placed in a small glass dish containing the egg. The idea is that one of them will penetrate the egg, fertilizing it. On this occasion, however, for some unknown reason fertilization did not take place. Nothing further could be done. The disappointed couple went home.

The Brennans' third attempt, in November, was even less successful. Jan underwent the operation for egg removal (known as a laparoscopy) but she had already ovulated and there was no egg to be found. They went back again in June 1980. This time an egg was collected, and to the Brennans' delight, when the sperm was put with it, fertilization did take place.

Now it was necessary to wait two or three days, while the embryo developed. By the end of the first day, the two nuclei—the genetic heart of the egg and of the sperm—had fused together. Another six hours and the single cell thus formed had split into two. About ten hours later each of these cells had divided, resulting in a cluster of four cells. At this stage Leeton transferred the embryo into Jan's womb. This was done by pushing a thin tube through her vagina, and then injecting the embryo, in a little fluid, down the tube.

Then began the waiting period. Would the embryo embed in the lining of her womb? It takes several days before tests can be carried out to see if pregnancy has occurred. When the results came, they were negative. Jan was not pregnant.

In October 1980 the Brennans went through the whole

procedure again. By this time the Monash team was using a fertility drug to stimulate ovulation, so that women on the programme would produce more than one egg at a time, and thus have a greater chance of at least one embryo surviving. Jan had taken the drug, and Leeton was able to obtain two eggs from the laparoscopy. Both were fertilized successfully, and both were transferred to Jan's womb. Again she had to wait for the tests. This time they were positive. She was pregnant, with twins.

The Brennans were, as Jan put it, 'grinning from ear to ear each time we looked at each other'; but their worries were still not over. During the eighth week of pregnancy, Jan found she was losing blood. An ultrasound scan showed that one of the twins had died. Jan rested in hospital for eight days, and then went nervously home. At fourteen weeks there was more bleeding, more anxiety, and another spell in hospital. Fortunately no damage had occurred. On 23 July 1981, just three years and a dozen IVF babies after the birth of Louise Brown, Pippin Brennan was born. She weighed 3.2 kilograms (7 lb.), and had auburn hair and blue eyes.

Despite the early disappointments, the Brennans' story is an IVF triumph. In the interests of balance, we should tell a different story.

Like Jan Brennan, Isabel Bainbridge's reproductive problems began when she was nineteen. After many bouts of appendicitis she had her appendix removed. During the operation it was noted that a cyst on one of her ovaries had recently ruptured. The ensuing complications left her with blocked Fallopian tubes. Later, when she married, she had painful medical treatment over many months to dissolve the tissue blocking the tubes. Then a test to see if the treatment had been successful caused a serious infection in both tubes. Eighteen months later she had an operation to repair the tubes but still she did not become pregnant. As a result of the unresolved tensions caused by her unsuccessful attempts to become pregnant, Isabel's first marriage broke down. By this time Isabel had been told by her doctor that she would be unlikely ever to become pregnant.

During the time between her first and second marriage Isabel became unexpectedly pregnant but the pregnancy turned out to be ectopic, and had to be terminated. She was told there was no chance of ever becoming pregnant again as the remaining tube appeared to be severely damaged; but within a year she was pregnant again and once again it was ectopic.

When Isabel remarried, she and her husband Toby were considered by the adoption agencies to be too old, at thirty-five, to parent a healthy, new-born baby. It was suggested that they might be considered suitable to adopt a mentally retarded or physically handicapped child. Neither of them considered this to be a suitable alternative to the normal healthy family they were hoping to have. Isabel returned to her gynaecologist who recommended either one final attempt at tubal repair or IVF treatment. As a nursing sister at the Royal Women's Hospital in Melbourne, she knew of the experimental IVF programme being developed by Ian Johnston, who was at that time working with Carl Wood. Because the work was still so new and had had no success at that time, Isabel and Toby chose the tubal repair work first. Isabel's last ectopic pregnancy had not entered the Fallopian tube but had grown on, and later torn off, the end of the tube, leaving it intact although still twisted and blocked. Again the treatment failed to result in the wanted pregnancy. Another year passed before the couple approached Johnston and asked to be put on the IVF programme. Isabel had her first laparoscopy in April 1978 and an egg was obtained but Toby found it impossible to masturbate under such stressful circumstances, and so fertilization could not be attempted.

Isabel's next laparoscopy was in August 1979. An egg was obtained, and Toby was able to produce the required sperm. The egg fertilized, and the embryo was transferred to Isabel's womb. Anxiously she and Toby waited for the results of the tests. They were negative.

In November Isabel was ready for another laparoscopy. When she reached hospital, however, it was found that she was already ovulating, and she was sent home. A month later she was back again, underwent laparoscopy, had an egg removed, fertilized, and transferred to the womb, but again the embryo did not implant. In May 1980 she had her fourth laparoscopy, an egg was obtained and fertilized but then accidentally lost in the laboratory. In September 1980 she was prepared for laparoscopy again but was sent home when it became evident that there was an error in the results of her urine tests.

By this time Ian Johnston and Carl Wood were working separately, and the Bainbridges decided to switch teams. So Isabel had her fifth laparoscopy with Wood's team in October 1981. All went well. An embryo resulted, and was transferred. The initial tests were positive. For ten days Isabel seemed to be pregnant. Then she had a heavy period, which may have been an early spontaneous abortion. Afterwards the tests were negative.

The Bainbridges were still under forty. They could have tried again; but gradually over the next year they decided that they would not. Isabel describes this decision as coming to an agreement with herself that she couldn't stand any more pain of the sort that she had been going through. She had been trying to become pregnant in one way or another for seventeen years. Now she wanted to close that chapter of her life, and do something else. She began to realize that there was another way out: acceptance of infertility and therefore choosing child-free living. At first, she and Toby were not sure if they could cope with this prospect; but by the beginning of 1983, they were getting on with their new lives, and starting to enjoy doing the kinds of things that are difficult or impossible for couples with children.

For the Bainbridges, IVF was no triumph. Instead it brought much pain and disappointment. Nevertheless they do not regret having gone through the process. As Isabel put it:

> I knew I had to experience infertility from the beginning to the end, even the depressions and the misery of feeling those emotions. I knew that it was some special part of my life. I didn't like it but I had to go through that stage of my life.
>
> Coming to terms with infertility and learning to live past it has challenged my life in a way which no pregnancy or child could ever have done for me.

How well does it work?

We have seen that for some couples, like the Brennans, IVF succeeds in producing the baby they want; for others, like the Bainbridges, it does not. Which is the more typical result? How often does an IVF treatment lead to a child?

Before we get into the figures, there are a couple of points to be noted. First, it would be unrealistic to expect every treatment to produce a child. That would be a far higher standard for IVF than occurs under natural conditions. Studies of healthy young women engaging in frequent sexual intercourse without contraception indicate that a pregnancy occurs only once in every three or four monthly cycles. By and large this is not, as one might imagine, due to an absence of fertilization. The egg can be fertilized, and the sperm remain viable, over a two- or three-day period, so sexual intercourse two or three times a week is usually enough to ensure fertilization. The reason pregnancy does not occur more often is that many of the newly created embryos fail to implant in the womb. Instead they are washed down the vagina, too tiny even to be noticed. There is evidence that many of these embryos are abnormal, so this may be a natural method of screening out embryos that would otherwise result in grossly defective offspring.

Edwards has suggested that IVF might eventually reach a higher success rate than natural reproduction, for two reasons. First, it is possible to verify that fertilization has taken place. Second, it is possible to check that the embryo is dividing in an apparently normal manner before putting it back. These tests for normality will no doubt improve still further. So Edwards believes a success rate of one pregnancy for every two embryo transfers is attainable. But even a success rate of one birth for every four treatments would not compare too badly with the natural rate.

Secondly, when success rates are discussed, it is important to be clear how the figures are expressed. One can talk of the number of pregnancies obtained, or the number of live births. Spontaneous abortions or miscarriages occur both in natural reproduction and in IVF. There are further complications: the success rate can be expressed as a ratio of pregnancies (or births) per patient seen over, say, a three-year period, or as pregnancies (or births) per individual treatment (that is, per laparoscopy), or per egg obtained (the number of eggs obtained from a single laparoscopy varies from none to a dozen or more), or per egg fertilized, or per embryo transferred to the womb. Obviously the way you want the success rate expressed will vary according to your interest in the programme. An infertile couple wondering about their chances of having a child by IVF will want to know the number of patients who, over some period of time like three years, actually give birth to a child. A right-to-life organization, concerned about the fate of embryos, would be more interested in the success rate per egg fertilized. Scientists seeking to improve the treatment could be interested in any of the figures, but they most often talk about the number of pregnancies per laparoscopy.

So what are the figures? The most successful IVF centres—in Cambridge, England; Melbourne, Australia; and the first American centre, in Norfolk, Virginia—now have a pregnancy per laparoscopy rate of 15–25 per cent. This means that they obtain one pregnancy for each four, five, or six egg collections they carry out—which may not sound very high but is getting close to the natural rate of one pregnancy per three or four cycles. Remember, too, that patients can have more than one laparoscopy—the Melbourne teams, for example, normally allow three tries before a couple must go back to the end of the queue. Thus patients who get to the egg collection stage have a better than a fifty-fifty chance of getting pregnant from one of their three egg collections. Naturally the odds drop if we include in the figures those patients who do not get to this stage—for example, women who are found not to be ovulating. We should also note that about 20 per cent of established IVF pregnancies end in spontaneous abortion—a rate that is not higher than that for normal reproduction, once the greater average age of IVF patients is taken into account.

Another relevant comparison is with the success rate of surgical attempts to repair damaged Fallopian tubes. Before IVF, this was the most common method of attempting to overcome this form of infertility. It succeeds in no more than 30 per cent of patients—and this figure does not include women like Jan Brennan, who was not even considered for surgery because her tubes had been removed entirely. Thus IVF can now claim to be nearly as successful a method of treatment as tubal surgery; and in addition it is able to help some patients who cannot be helped by surgery.

If we try to measure how many of the embryos created by IVF eventually make it through to birth, the story becomes more complex. With the more successful centres, between a quarter and a third of all transfers result in a pregnancy—but these higher rates are often based on the transfer of more than one embryo. One trial carried out in Melbourne resulted in a pregnancy rate of 12 per cent when only one embryo was put into the uterus, but rates of 28 per cent from the transfer of two embryos, and 40 per cent from the transfer of three. Thus the survival rate *per embryo* transferred is much lower than the pregnancy rate *per transfer operation*, and is generally in the order of 12–18 per cent. Even this figure, however, is not necessarily an indication of the percentage of all created embryos that survive. As we have seen, a single egg collection may result in from none to a dozen ripe eggs being collected. To allay opposition on ethical grounds, some centres, such as the one in Norfolk, Virginia, will fertilize only as many eggs as the patient is willing to have transferred to her womb; others, like Carl Wood's team in Melbourne, have fertilized all suitable eggs and selected the best one, two, or three (depending on the wishes of the patient) for transfer. The remaining normal embryos have been frozen, in preference to simply being thrown out. Since the survival rate for frozen embryos is, so far, very low, for the purpose of calculating the survival rate these frozen embryos could be numbered among those that do not survive.

Wood's approach may result in a higher birth rate per egg collection, because of the greater availability of embryos from which to select those considered most likely to grow normally. At the same time it will result in a lower rate of births per embryo created, because so many more embryos are created. According to figures supplied by Dr Alan Trounson, between the beginning of 1980 and February 1982 Wood's team obtained 876 eggs from 272 patients, and succeeded in fertilizing 633 of them. These 633 embryos produced 45 live births. Thus fourteen embryos were created for every one that finally became a baby. Whether this loss of embryonic life matters is something we shall discuss in the next chapter.

Who wants it?

The next question we shall ask is: How many people are there who are likely to use IVF? On how big a scale is the treatment likely to be employed?

To answer this, the first thing we need to know is how many infertile couples there are, and how many of these couples have a strong desire to have children. It, has been estimated that infertility is a problem for at least 10 per cent of all married couples. In perhaps 30 per cent of these cases, the cause of infertility is a defect in the Fallopian tubes. This is, as we have seen, the kind of defect which IVF was specifically designed to overcome. There may also be other forms of infertility which can be successfully treated by IVF. Certainly the Melbourne IVF teams have had success in treating cases of infertility in which the cause of the problem was not known and did not appear to be tubal damage.

Some women who are infertile because of defective tubes can be treated by microsurgery. In fact, in the United States somewhere between 15,000 and 30,000 operations to repair defective tubes are carried out each year (about 10 per cent of these operations are attempts to reverse an earlier voluntary sterilization). But as we have already said, many women cannot be helped by tubal surgery. Dr Howard Jones and Dr Georgeanna Jones, who founded the first United States IVF centre, in Norfolk, had previously worked for thirty-five years at Johns Hopkins University, specializing in the treatment of infertility. As Dr Georgeanna Jones has said: 'We had more or less accepted that there were, say, 15 per cent of patients for whom we could do nothing. Those with severe tubal problems, blockages, or difficulties that led to the Fallopian tubes being removed altogether. Then, we came to Norfolk . . .'

Even in the case of women who are reasonable prospects for surgery, IVF would probably be preferred if it offered comparable success rates. Tubal surgery involves a much more major operation for the women. It also carries a significant risk of one major complication—an ectopic pregnancy. There does not appear to be any comparable risk for IVF. (We discuss the question of safety in more detail in the next chapter.)

If we look beyond the most standard form of IVF, we open the door to an even larger potential demand. For example, the use of eggs donated by another woman would enable women who are not ovulating to become pregnant and experience childbirth. Transfer of an embryo into the womb of another woman, who would act as a surrogate for the genetic mother until the child was born, would enable a woman who had no womb to have a child that was genetically hers. (It could also enable any woman who could afford it to avoid the inconvenience of pregnancy by hiring someone else for the job.) But we shall not explore the numbers of people who might wish to make use of these possibilities.

If we revert to the potential demand for standard IVF, it is clear that a very large number of people may wish to use the treatment. Clifford Grobstein's Science and Public Policy research team at the University of California, San Diego, has estimated that in the United States there may be some 740,000 couples interested in IVF. Figures for other nations would probably be roughly similar, in proportion to their population.

Figures of this sort are for the total population who are infertile and in the age bracket at which they are likely to want to reproduce—for women, this is generally taken as between twenty-four and thirty-six years of age. Because IVF has not previously been available, all the women in this age group who are anxious to use IVF could be expected to want to use it immediately. Hence there is an enormous backlog of potential users. If IVF becomes sufficiently readily available for all those who want it to be able to have it, the annual demand would fall dramatically. If we assume that each couple would want to have two children over the twelve-year period in which the woman is between twenty-four and thirty-six, the annual demand would be one-sixth of the total number of couples wanting the treatment at some point during these years. In the United States, this would amount to a little over 123,000.

One way of reducing this annual demand would be to attempt to provide twins for all couples seeking two children. IVF programmes which implant two or three embryos are already producing twins at about ten times the natural rate, and most childless couples are delighted to find that they have not one, but two children. This is especially true of older women, who may not have another opportunity for a second child. Not everyone, however, would be equally happy with twins, and some younger couples could well reject this short cut to a larger family.

There are, of course, many factors that reduce this demand. As we saw from Jan Brennan's account, the procedure is not an easy one, and there is no guarantee of success. That alone would deter some couples. There is also the financial cost to the patient, which we shall be discussing shortly. Here it is enough to say that even when the full cost is born by the patient and cannot be recovered from health insurance funds—as is the case, for example, at the Norfolk IVF centre—the demand for the service is still overwhelming. The Norfolk centre was designed to handle about 200 patients a year. Following publicity from their first birth, the centre received more than 6,000 inquiries. In Melbourne, where there is less of a cost deterrent, Wood's team has a waiting-list of about 2,000 couples and couples can expect to wait about three years before their turn comes. The ethical objections to IVF which have been expressed by the Roman Catholic Church do not appear to have a major effect on demand. In Australia, where 25 per cent of the population is Roman Catholic and the Church's criticisms of the programme have received wide publicity, Catholics remain on the waiting-list in numbers proportionate to their numbers in the population as a whole. Len Brennan, for example, describes himself as a practising Catholic. We administered a questionnaire to a sample of couples on Carl Wood's IVF programme, and found that 22 per cent of our sample described themselves as Roman Catholic.

In this section we have set out to answer the question of how many people may want to use IVF. We have not attempted to assess the strength of their desire, or whether it is a desire that we ought to try to satisfy. These questions will be tackled in the next chapter.

How much does it cost?

IVF is an expensive procedure, but, by current medical standards, not extraordinarily so. The Royal Women's Hospital in Melbourne reckons the cost at about \$A1,740 per laparoscopy and embryo transfer. This does not include any allowance for the preliminary investigations which all infertile couples must have, or for any social work or counselling. It is therefore a conservative estimate, and the real cost is probably somewhere between \$A2,000 and \$A4,000. The largest single item in the cost is five days in hospital, but there are many other tests and procedures which make up the total.

In the Australian health system, almost everyone belongs to a government-subsidized health insurance fund, which reimburses medical expenses. Australian health insurance funds do not specifically cover the costs of IVF; they do, however, cover the costs of hospitalization and of several other procedures, such as the laparoscopy, which are part of the IVF treatment. Thus Australian patients end up paying about $A800 for each cycle of treatment. The rest is reimbursed by their health insurance.

In the United States, medical costs are generally higher and health insurance less comprehensive. IVF is no exception. For IVF treatment in Norfolk, patients are charged $1,650 for a preliminary screening procedure, and then another $3,100 for each laparoscopy for egg collection—a total of $4,750. At present most US health insurance funds are refusing to cover this cost, on the grounds that the procedure is experimental. This may change as the procedure establishes itself.

In Britain, Edwards and Steptoe have set up a private clinic at Bourn Hall, near Cambridge. The cost to patients here is similar to that in Norfolk, around £2,000, but the British private health insurance fund will cover the costs of some of their members. Elsewhere in Britain, one or two centres are offering IVF on the National Health Service, at no cost to the patients.

To put this in perspective, a comparison with the cost of surgery to repair damaged tubes is helpful. In the United States, if the damage is minor and can be repaired by normal surgical techniques, the cost—including both hospital charges and the surgeon's fees—is around $4,000. If the problem is more complicated and requires microsurgery, the cost would exceed $6,500. For the reversal of a sterilization operation, the higher figure would apply. Of course, if the operation is successful the woman should be able to conceive as many children as she desires, whereas for IVF the cost must be incurred for each pregnancy. Still, it is clear that as long as the IVF success rates per laparoscopy are not too far behind the success rates for the tubal surgery, IVF is, in strictly economic terms, a reasonable alternative to more conventional methods of overcoming infertility.

These figures make no allowance for the cost of the research needed to develop IVF to its present stage. This cost is more difficult to assess. Clearly all those now providing IVF owe something to the pioneering work of Edwards and Steptoe. In 1971 Edwards and Steptoe applied to the British Medical Research Council for a grant to carry out experimental work on IVF in humans. They were refused, on the grounds that too few animal studies had been conducted. They went ahead anyway, without specific government funding. Similarly, in the United States, no government money at all has been spent on IVF, because the government has not been prepared to risk the political opposition of those who are against the procedure. It appears that private foundations have not funded IVF research within America either.

Only in Australia do we have even rough estimates of the research costs. During the developmental stage, when there was only one IVF group in Melbourne, the team received about one million Australian dollars in research grants from various sources. One of the largest grants came from the Ford Foundation, which provided money for research in reproductive biology that, by enabling us to learn how fertilization takes place, might also enable us to find better methods of contraception. Such by-products of IVF have yet to come to fruition, but the possibility remains that the research done for IVF will have other benefits as well.

One million dollars is a substantial sum. Again, however, if we see it in terms of the total cost of medical research it becomes a less dramatic figure. The United States spends an estimated *ten billion* dollars on medical research each year. In Australia research spending per head of population is much lower, but the National Health and Medical Research Council alone still provides $A18.7 m. per year.

What does the public think?

Might does not make right. Nor does public opinion. There are too many examples of morally outrageous practices which have had the support of a majority of the society which has practised them. That is why we are presenting the results of public-opinion surveys on IVF in this chapter, which sets out relevant facts about IVF, rather than in the next chapter, which discusses the ethical arguments. We should know what the majority think, but we should not feel in any way compelled to agree.

The first public-opinion polls on IVF were taken in the United States, in August 1978. Both Harris and Gallup conducted polls, each based on a sample of 1,500 people. The Harris poll interviewed women only, while Gallup interviewed both men and women. The polls were taken shortly after the much publicized birth of Louise Brown, and the Gallup poll showed that 93 per cent of their samples had heard or read about the birth.

The polls indicated clear majority approval of IVF as a means of helping couples who could not otherwise have children. The Gallup poll put the question in the following manner:

Some people oppose this type of operation because they feel it is 'not natural'. Other people favour it because it allows a husband and wife to have a child they could not otherwise have. Which point of view comes closer to your own?

Sixty per cent said they were in favour, 27 per cent opposed the operation, and the remaining 13 per cent had no opinion.

The Harris poll gave rise to some curious findings: on a general question about approval of the procedure, only 52 per cent approved, with 24 per cent disapproving and an equal number undecided. Yet 85 per cent of the sample were prepared to agree that the procedure should be available to married couples who are otherwise unable to have children. This suggests that the inclusion of the word 'married' and a reference to the inability to have children prompts a more favourable response than a general question about 'approval of the procedure'.

Some of the findings of the Harris poll sound a note of caution: 63 per cent agreed with the idea that IVF should be banned until further testing assured that it was not causing birth defects. Yet a majority—a bare 50 per cent—also agreed with a ban on federal government support of research into IVF: 42 per cent opposed such a ban.

The women were asked if they personally would use the method if they were unable to have a baby: 48 per cent said they would; 44 per cent said they would not. Significantly, willingness to use the method was higher—62 per cent—among women who were planning to have children. Asked if they preferred adoption or IVF as a means of having a child, 57 per cent said adoption, 21 per cent IVF, and 16 per cent were indifferent.

The Harris poll also asked some more specific questions which are related to some of the points raised in this book. Firstly, in contrast to the 85 per cent who accepted the procedure for married couples unable to have children, only 21 per cent thought it should be available to unmarried couples who are living together and unable to have children. This figure is a little less than the figure (22 per cent) of those who thought it should be available to single women who are unable to have children. (The difference is puzzling, but may reflect the idea that the unmarried couple are living in sin, whereas the test-tube method enables a single woman to have a child without having sexual intercourse.) Only 11 per cent thought that the procedure should be available to lesbians or homosexuals. (It is not clear what difference the addition of 'or homosexuals' was understood to make. Was it a reference to homosexual males? If so, was it envisaged that the homosexual would fertilize an egg to be implanted in a surrogate mother who would surrender it to the male homosexual? It would obviously have been better to treat lesbians and male homosexuals separately, since lesbians would not require the use of a surrogate.)

More women than not, by 49 per cent to 40 per cent, believed that where the husband is unable to provide healthy sperm, a married couple should be allowed to use donor sperm.

Finally, those surveyed were asked if they would allow doctors to remove more than one egg from a woman, fertilize them all, and then discard all but the one to be inserted for development: 45 per cent said they would allow this, 40 per cent said they would not, and 14 per cent were unsure. Disapproval of the discarding of the fertilized eggs was higher, but still not overwhelming, among Catholics: 39 per cent of Catholics said they would allow the additional eggs to be discarded, 48 per cent said they would not, and 12 per cent were unsure.

The Australian public has been more thoroughly surveyed on this issue than the public in any other country. The Roy Morgan Research Centre conducted polls in June 1981, February 1982, July 1982, and April 1983. The first two polls were based on a sample of 1,600 respondents; the last two on approximately 1,000. Different samples were used for each poll. In all four polls, public awareness of what was described as 'the test-tube baby method for helping married couples who can't have children' was very high—at least 92 per cent had heard of the method. Approval was also high—77 per cent in the first poll, dropping to 69 per cent in the middle two and climbing back to 74 per cent in the most recent one. No more than 13 per cent disapproved in any poll, the remainder being undecided

Having expressed an attitude, people were then asked: 'Why especially do you feel that way?' The most popular reply among those who approved was that it gives people the opportunity to have children. Others said that it was preferable to, or easier than, adoption, while another common reply was that the decision is up to the parents. Among those who disapproved, the reason most often given was that it is unnatural. Only 2 per cent of all respondents gave religious grounds for disapproving.

The people surveyed were then told that at present married couples who have the test-tube-baby treatment have to pay $A350 (*sic*) per treatment, and that about one treatment in eight has been successful in producing a baby. They were then asked if couples should be able to claim the treatment on health insurance. A minimum of 64 per cent replied that they should, with about 20 per cent saying they should not, and the remainder undecided.

A more detailed analysis of the responses shows that people over fifty were much less likely to approve than those in their twenties (60 per cent approval as compared with 86 per cent) and those who completed secondary schooling had a much higher rate of approval than those who did not (78 per cent for those with tertiary education as compared with only 47 per cent for those who had only primary education).

Religious affiliation made less difference than might have been expected. Roman Catholics approved of the method almost as frequently (67 per cent) as those who said they had no religion (73 per cent). Anglicans were more approving still (79 per cent) while those professing a non-Christian religion—presumably mostly Moslem or Jewish—had the lowest rate of approval (61 per cent).

The poll carried out in July 1982 was different from the others in two respects. First, in addition to the straightforward question on the use of IVF to help married couples who can't have children, it also asked about embryo freezing, surrogate mothers, and embryo donation. To avoid bombarding our readers with too many figures all at once, we shall set out the responses to these questions when we come to the issues with which they deal.

The second special feature of the third poll was that it was an international one. Identical questions were put to a sample of 936 people in Britain. Britons were as aware of the test-tube baby method as Australians. With 62 per cent approving and 20 per cent disapproving, they were only slightly less positive than Australians about the method as a means of helping married couples who can't have children.

In summary, polls carried out in the United States, Australia, and Britain all show clear approval of IVF when used to help infertile married couples. The lowest approval rating in any poll was 60 per cent and the highest disapproval rating 27 per cent, both in the United States Gallup poll. We repeat that this says nothing about whether IVF is an ethically sound procedure. To this question we shall now turn.

2 IVF; THE SIMPLE CASE

In March 1982, when the Melbourne team led by Carl Wood was turning *in vitro* fertilization from a miraculous experiment into a routine treatment, the state government of Victoria—the state which has Melbourne as its capital—announced that it would establish a committee to investigate the social, ethical, and legal issues surrounding IVF. The announcement no doubt has much to do with the fact that a state election was about to be held, and the Roman Catholic Archbishop of Melbourne has expressed concern about the whole 'test-tube baby' programme. If that was the motive, the ploy failed. The government was defeated. Its successor nevertheless honoured the pledge, set up the Committee, and told it to make an interim report within three months. Faced with the impossible task of resolving within three months the host of complex social, ethical, and legal issues surrounding IVF, the Committee ruthlessly pruned away one tricky issue after another, until it was dealing with the simplest possible case of IVF: the case of the married, infertile couple, where the egg is taken from the wife and the sperm from the husband, and the embryo or embyros created are all inserted into the womb of the wife.

Using this narrow focus, the Committee was able to avoid, in its interim report, issues like IVF for unmarried couples or for single women; the use of donated sperm, eggs, or embryos; and the disposal of surplus embryos. We think the strategy adopted by the Victorian Committee a happy one because it separated the objections to IVF itself from the many other objections that apply to some applications of IVF, or to some ways of carrying out IVF, but not to all. Therefore in the present chapter we consider only those argument that challenge the simple case of IVF, as described in the preceding paragraph. We shall set aside all other arguments until the next chapter. Even the crucial question of the moral status of the embryo will be postponed, for that objection has little relevance in a situation in which every embryo created is given all the assistance within our power to enable it to grow to a child.

Doing what comes unnaturally

In the previous chapter, when looking at public opinion polls on IVF, we quoted the question the Gallup organization put to its American sample:

Some people oppose this type of operation because they feel it is 'not natural'. Other people favour it because it allows a husband and wife to have a child they could not otherwise have. Which point of view comes closer to your own?

Presumably whoever devised that question felt that 'it is not natural' was the best way of summing up the disquiet many people feel about IVF. As we saw, more than a quarter of the sample said that this attitude was closer to their own than the alternative more favourable attitude. But in what sense is IVF really 'not natural'? And what does it matter, anyway?

When John Stuart Mill wrote his essay 'Nature', he began by saying that although words like 'nature' and 'natural' have 'at all times filled a great place in the thoughts and taken a strong hold on the feelings of mankind', they have 'become entangled in so many foreign associations, mostly of a very powerful and tenacious character' that they are now 'one of the most copious sources of false taste, false philosophy, false morality, and even bad law'. In following the debate over IVF, we have found that the words Mill wrote in the middle of the nineteenth century still accurately describe the use made today of appeals to what is natural; and we recommend to the interested reader Mill's clear and full exposure of the errors made in such appeals. All we can do in the present section is set out briefly some of the ambiguities and fallacies in the argument that IVF is wrong because it is 'unnatural'.

The constantly recurring objection that IVF—and indeed biotechnology in general—is unnatural is raised by a wide variety of people in a wide variety of ways—some crude, others extremely subtle. The cruder versions are generally advanced by people who are not aware that what is and what is not natural is no straightforward matter of fact. It is a complex philosophical question. We will discuss a number of the varieties of the 'unnaturalness' objection, starting with the most simple-minded version.

Let us call the first version of the objection the 'descriptive' view. It holds that what is natural is what occurs in nature untouched by human intervention. Nature is, on the descriptive view, the world apart from human beings. Since IVF does not occur except by human intervention, it is therefore (on this view) not natural. However, by the same token, neither is any other form of medical treatment. The opponent of IVF would have to reject all forms of medical treatment.

Behind this version of the objection to interfering with nature may lie the notion that the normal or natural course of events is a benign one, and hence we ought not to seek to alter it. But nature is not benign. Nature—the course of events that we do not control—is blind to the welfare of any creature. The laws of physics, of chemistry, of biology, and of evolution have no care for whether children starve to death in famines or animals perish miserably in droughts. It is therefore monstrous to believe that we should leave the world alone, meekly suffering the consequences without daring to challenge the 'natural' course of events.

This point is so conclusive that it is hard to believe that more than a handful of people really object to IVF because it is unnatural in this sense. More perhaps object to IVF on the grounds that it is unnatural in another, though still descriptive, sense. There is another sense of 'natural' which means something like 'occurring in the normal course of events'. For instance, we say things like: 'Demands for wage increases are a natural result of rapidly increasing prices', and 'When Jill told Jack she would be home for dinner, and was still not home by 10 p.m., it was natural that he should be worried.' So a more plausible version of the descriptive view would be to say that IVF is unnatural because it does not happen in the normal course of things.

This version may be plausible, but it is not an effective criticism of IVF or anything else to say that it does not happen in the normal course of events. IVF is an innovation, and it is true of every innovation that it does not happen in the normal course of events. Of course somebody could say that they just don't like innovations, and they prefer things which do happen in the normal course of events. But they could not possibly mean it. In the normal course of events people diagnosed as suffering from an advanced cancer will not recover. But sometimes they do. It would be hard to imagine anyone regretting this departure from the normal course of events, whether or not the recovery resulted from innovative medical treatment.

The opponent of IVF could say that the objection was not just that IVF is a departure from any normal course of events: the point is that this particular normal course of events—normal conception—has a unique value apart from the fact that it is the way things usually are done. But having said that, the objector would be changing ground. The objection would now no longer be on the grounds that IVF was 'unnatural', but rather on the grounds that 'normal' conception has unique value. This point however could wistfully be conceded by an infertile couple who wished to receive IVF treatment precisely because they could not achieve the 'unique value' of a 'normal' conception. A 'second best' method of conception may still be far better than none at all. Once the stigma has gone from the fact that IVF does not occur in the normal course of things, to point out that IVF is unnatural in the descriptive sense is to point out nothing which is at all damaging.

Another version of the unnaturalness objection is a claim put forward by some enthusiastic but unreflective members of the laity, though not by any clergy that we know of. It is the flat assertion that IVF is unnatural 'because it is not how God intended conception to occur'. The decisive question here is the obvious one—how do they know? Assuming the existence of a God who makes ordinations as to what is right and wrong, there is some difficulty in ascertaining this ordination on such a specific and technical matter as IVF. We cannot use past practices as a guide. God's will cannot be discovered by simply assuming that it is in accordance with the way things have always been done, since in that case, every innovation in history would have to be dismissed as contrary to God's will. In other words, every facet of our lives, which are after all governed by the sum of human innovations to date, would have to be denounced as a violation of the will of God. Observation of what has previously occurred will not, therefore, tell us what God is willing to have occur.

The alternative to deduction by observation is revelation. The difficulty here is that those upon whom God would most reasonably be expected to vouchsafe revelation, do not all seem to be in possession of the same information. There never has been unanimity among divines as to what exactly is the will of God. It already is clear that there will be no unanimity either on matters relating to biotechnology.

A further problem arises from the simple oddity of the suggestion that something may be contrary to the will of God and yet still occur. If God is (as He is agreed to be) all powerful, then it is extraordinary to suggest that IVF is contrary to His will. For surely He would then not allow IVF to develop. The reply of course will be that He could stop it if He wanted to, but He is just allowing us to exercise our free will, and thereby fall into sin. He is merely testing us. But then if God is all knowing, He would already know the results of our test. There is therefore little point in testing us. All in all, an objector who would have us believe that IVF is contrary to the will of God, is forced to give us a very unflattering account of Divine behaviour.

A much more subtle view is the suggestion that IVF is unnatural because it contravenes 'natural law'. Natural law theory is of very ancient origins, but has endured, in various forms, until the present day. It holds that over and above the laws which mortals make for themselves there is a coherent body of 'laws of nature' by reference to which human laws can be judged, and perhaps be found wanting in justice or some other necessary ingredient. These natural laws, as their name implies, are not grounded in the transitory needs of human beings or social systems, but in nature itself. The difficult question of course is how the laws of nature are to be identified, and different natural law theorists have given different answers. Some have held that the natural laws are laws of reason. They can be discovered by intuition, according to some, or by right-minded observation, according to others, or by reasoning without self-contradiction, according to another school. A different group of natural law thinkers has held that the laws of nature can be discovered by reference to a state of nature—perhaps a notional state of humankind (hypothetically) existing before the development of human societies, or perhaps—as with the *ius gentium* of the practically minded ancient Romans—by reference to the rules observed by right-minded citizens everywhere, even if they lacked the benefit of Roman law. Yet another (and in our opinion the most plausible) group of natural law thinkers have held that the laws of nature can be discovered by reference to the ends of natural things—the circumstances in which natural kinds flourish or achieve their fulfilment.

This last version of natural law theory owes much to Aristotle and to the Stoics, and has been held by many Catholic philosophers. The theory does not just say that human beings have a certain end which constitutes their flourishing. All things equally have an end, which is defined by their essence (for example the end of an acorn is to become an oak) and even human acts have an essence which defines the appropriate way in which they should be performed. It was on this strand of natural law theory that Pope Paul VI relied when he issued his encyclical banning artificial contraception. One of the strands in his argument was that the essence of the act of sexual intercourse was procreation of the species: consequently artificial contraception subverted the essence of the act and was therefore contrary to nature.

We have heard it argued informally by theologians that IVF is unnatural in exactly the sense in which the Pope declared contraception to be unnatural. The suggestion was that since the essence of sexual intercourse was procreation, to divorce procreation from the sexual act, by transferring it to the laboratory, is to subvert the essence of the act of sexual intercourse. But even someone who accepts the Pope's argument about contraception should not accept this attempt to run the argument backwards. If procreation were the essence of sexual intercourse, it might follow on some views of natural law that it was wrong to take steps which prevented the fulfilment of the essential goal of sexual intercourse; but how would it follow that when infertility prevented the achievement of this essential goal through sexual intercourse, it was wrong to achieve it in some other way? To take a parallel example, does the fact that nourishment is the essential goal of eating mean that a baby with a digestive problem should not be temporarily fed through a tube? If not, why should the essential goal of sexual intercourse be treated any differently?

Indeed we would say that those natural law doctrines which Catholic scholars have most enthusiastically embraced lead to the conclusion that IVF should be encouraged. Remember that it is not IVF that prevents sexual intercourse from achieving its essential goal of procreation. Accident or disease has already seen to that. IVF aims at restoring to the infertile person the possibility of procreation. If procreation is an essential human goal—we do not say it is, but this view fits well with a natural law outlook—then IVF helps people to achieve this goal. When people who desire children are prevented from reproducing, they are prevented from achieving the form of fulfilment or flourishing that they seek. So at least to the extent that biotechnology serves as a therapy for unwanted infertility, natural law theorists ought not merely to permit it: they ought to be among its strongest advocates.

To conclude this discussion, we ask again why human beings and their deeds should be regarded as separate from nature and opposed to it. Are we not ourselves part of nature? In designing ways of overcoming obstacles to the fulfilment of deep human desires, are we not acting with our own rational nature? On this, we leave the last word with the distinguished Protestant theologian and bioethicist, Joseph Fletcher:

Any attempt to set up an antinomy between natural and biologic reproduction, on the one hand, and artificial or designed reproduction, on the other, is absurd. The real choice is between accidental or random reproduction and rationally willed or chosen reproduction . . . laboratory reproduction is radically human compared to conception by ordinary heterosexual intercourse. It is willed, chosen, purposed and controlled, and surely those are among the traits that distinguish *Homo sapiens* from others in the animal genus, from the primates down.

Slipping towards Brave New World?

Aldous Huxley's celebrated novel *Brave New World* describes a society that most readers find repellent. The family has been abolished. Every human being is conceived in a test-tube and gestation takes place in a laboratory. At nine months they are not born, but 'decanted'. Infancy and childhood are spent communally, and words like 'motherhood' are regarded as obscene. During childhood everyone receives intensive brainwashing, day and night. At night children receive 'hypnopaedic sleep teaching': an insinuating voice, throughout their sleeping periods, gives them moral instruction. They are taught that promiscuity is a moral duty, that the quest for pleasure is the purpose of life, and that the world they live in can hardly be improved. A rigid hierarchical structure is maintained by genetic engineering. Society is divided into Alphas (the intellectual élite), Betas (people who can take secondary responsibility), and Gammas, Deltas, and Epsilons. Epsilons are semi-morons, genetically designed to do the most boring jobs without feeling frustrated. Only the Alphas and Betas are individual in appearance. The others are mass-produced by a system that has the same effect as cloning. A Gamma, a Delta, or an Epsilon may have ninety-odd identical siblings. Everyone, however, is conditioned to be supremely happy with her or his station in life, and to wish for no other.

Writing in 1932, Huxley set his novel in the year 682 After Ford—or 2629 by our reckoning. Later, in his foreword to the 1950 edition, he said that it could happen in one century. Many now believe that a society like the one Huxley described is much closer than that. In *Who Should Play God?*, a book discussing IVF, cloning, and genetic engineering, Ted Howard and Jeremy Rifkin predict a step-by-step, corporate-based private enterprise introduction of the new biotechnology:

Over a period of time (the next twenty-five to fifty years) the cumulative effect of this step-by-step process will be the emergence of a kind of corporate Brave New World, not unlike the one Huxley fantasized about over forty years ago. It is a much less dramatic approach to the ultimate enslavement of the human species, but the results are no less terrifying than if they had been ruthlessly imposed by some mad political dictator. The only real difference is that with this approach we will march passively and in some cases even willingly into this new reality without pain, without inconvenience, and without awareness.

The point Howard and Rifkin are making has also been made in countless newspaper stories and magazine articles about IVF and associated developments in baby-making. As early as 1965, when Robert Edwards published the results of his first attempts at ripening human eggs in a laboratory, the *Sunday Times* said the experiments were 'reminiscent of Aldous Huxley's *Brave New World*'. That refrain has been echoed with monotonous regularity ever since. The implication is that we had better stop these new developments right now, before it is too late. But how close is the connection between IVF and Huxley's society of the future?

Huxley described an advanced industrial society which had mastered artificial reproduction and genetic engineering. That, however, was not all. There was also extensive brainwashing, a rigid caste system, absence of all family ties, government-approved use of mind-altering drugs, and an absence of any real choice regarding one's way of living. The fact that we have not yet mastered artificial reproduction and genetic engineering is therefore not the only thing that distinguishes our society from Huxley's dystopia. Accordingly it is a mistake to think that advances in biotechnology will in themselves bring about that kind of society.

The most odious aspects of Huxley's world are undoubtedly its caste system and its lack of freedom. These have existed in many societies, and indeed still do exist in some, without any recourse to biotechnology. The human race does not need advanced biotechnology to aid it in developing odious social systems.

Since major advances in biotechnology are taking place all around us, it is more illuminating to consider the nature of the social systems in which these advances are occurring. The major IVF centres are in Australia, the United States, and Western Europe. Now whatever may be the defects of the social systems of those countries, they all subscribe to the principle of equality before the law. All hold democratic elections. Every adult has an equal vote. All allow free speech and freedom of assembly. All agree that the state exists to serve the citizen, rather than the other way round. However defectively these ideals are given effect, they are widely respected, and embedded in constitutional, legal, political, and social practices.

Our question then is this: 'Will the advances taking place in biotechnology in (for example) Melbourne in 1983, make that city more like Huxley's London in the year 682 After Ford?' The answer is that a lot of things which appear to have no relationship to biotechnology would have to change before it would. The Brave New World's caste system could hardly appear without the sweeping away of all sorts of constitutional and political restraints which guarantee citizens' equality in certain respects. Any Huxleyan programme to do away with the family would be unlikely to get off the ground. (The chances of introducing an hallucinogen like Huxley's soma, in the place of alcohol, as the officially sanctioned mind-altering drug, also seem slight.) Advances in biotechnology alone will not plunge us irrevocably into the depths of Huxley's nightmare. A technology is only a tool. How a society chooses to use a tool will be influenced by the characteristics of the society in question. In the societies with which we are here concerned, there are deeply embedded obstacles to the pursuit of Huxleyan programmes.

The matter, however, cannot be allowed to rest there. What we have said so far is too superficial. We have to recognize that a tool can have effects beyond its narrow use. Societies utilize technologies, but technologies also affect the structure of the societies using them. Consider another new technology: the microchip. This technology enables typing pools to be replaced with a word processor and retail staff to be replaced by a check-out clerk with a computerized till which simultaneously registers purchases, orders new stock from the warehouse, and puts a replacement procedure in motion. The technology dramatically reduces the number of people employed in the clerical, retail, entertainment, and communications industries. The seriousness of this effect is increased by the fact that these people usually do not have other jobs to go to. The technology also provides the capacity for greater surveillance of those workers who remain. The same technology which does away with several mechanical typewriters (and human typists) and replaces them with a single video display unit attached to a computer, can as easily record the number of times the operator presses the button, or even the content of telephone conversation between executives. In other words microchip technology leads to a fundamental shift in the work place—a shift towards greater surveillance and tighter central control.

Whatever our attitude to these various changes, it is evident that microchip technology is not just a neutral tool: it is clearly society-forming as well as society-formed. It is a tool which contributes to the future shape of the society which utilizes it.

Is biotechnology like microchip technology in that its use will inevitably have major society-forming effects? If it is, then what becomes of our suggestion that the political and social obstacles to society developing on Huxleyan lines are enough to ensure that we can easily have the new biotechnology without having a Brave New World? Is that suggestion not undercut by the fact that technologies do change societies?

We think that in the simplest case of IVF, at least, the answer to these questions is clear: the new technology will not alter the social system at all. In the simplest case, the IVF parents are as much the parents of their children as any parents possibly can be. This technology, applied in this manner, does not bring Brave New World any closer at all.

To this claim we can anticipate a familiar reply: the Slippery Slope Argument. In the context of IVF, this argument has been put most strongly by Dr Leon Kass, in a paper commissioned by the Ethics Advisory Board of the United States Department of Health, Education and Welfare. In September 1978 the Board had been asked to consider whether the United States Government should fund research into IVF. Kass argued that it should not, and his paper made explicit the argument that the logic used to justify IVF for infertile married couples 'knows no boundary'. Archly reversing the usual metaphor, he said: 'Once the genies let the babies into the bottle, it may be impossible to get them out again.' In summary, Kass argued against government funding for any research on IVF, one of his reasons being that 'it will be difficult to forestall dangerous present and future applications of this research and its logical extensions'.

In another paper presented to the Ethics Advisory Board, the philosopher Samuel Gorovitz replied to Kass's argument. Drawing on his experience as a skier, Gorovitz reminded the Board that it is possible to make judgements about which slippery slopes one can handle and which one cannot: 'It is a question of control and, in part, of judgment.' There is no reason, he said, to take seriously a view that implies a total absence of any control over future developments. We have the capacity to exercise judgement and control, we have exercised it on other issues in the past—liberalized abortion has not led to the selective slaughter of anyone in social disfavour—and we shall be able to exercise it in the future on this issue too.

Summing up this debate in his book *From Chance to Purpose*, Clifford Grobstein has drawn attention to the crucial role played by our purposes. If our purpose in developing IVF is simply to alleviate infertility in marriage due to blocked tubes, then no sanction has been given for anything that goes beyond this situation. If our purpose is broader, we may be on a slope that will take us further. What we have to do, Grobstein suggests, is spell out clearly what our purposes are, and how far we are willing to go. Each new issue that is outside our original purpose must then be considered afresh.

We agree with Grobstein that the limited purpose of carrying out IVF to assist married infertile couples—especially within the tight constraints of the simplest case—means that no precedent is set for the more far-reaching developments that might bring Brave New World appreciably closer. To continue the skiing metaphor, IVF in the simplest case is a beginners' playground that we can handle without much trouble. Whether other applications of IVF might put us on steeper and more dangerous slopes is something we shall discuss in later chapters.

How big a risk?

At a symposium on 'fabricated babies' held in Washington, DC in 1971, one of the speakers was James Watson, who had won the Nobel Prize for his discovery of the double helix structure of DNA, the molecule governing heredity. Robert Edwards was also present, and Watson addressed him directly: 'You can only go ahead with your work,' he said, 'if you accept the necessity of infanticide. There are going to be a lot of mistakes. What are you going to do with the mistakes?' Another speaker at the symposium was Paul Ramsay, Professor of Theology at Princeton University. Ramsey argued that the anticipated production of at least some deformed or retarded children during the early stages of IVF made it absolutely immoral to continue this research. Ramsey's views were published the following year in the highly respected

Journal of the American Medical Association. His conclusions were supported by Leon Kass, a third speaker at the symposium. 'It doesn't matter how many times the baby is tested while in the mother's womb,' said Kass, 'they will never be certain the baby won't be born without a defect.' Kass was also soon to put this view into print, in *The Public Interest.* Even a 1975 study by the prestigious United States National Research Council, *Assessing Biomedical Technologies,* concluded that the risk of mental retardation or other damage was too great for IVF ever to be tried.

Those working on IVF, like Edwards in England and Landrum Shettles in the United States, replied that there was data drawn from several animal species which indicated that IVF did not produce deformed offspring. The transfer of embryos was, as we saw in the previous chapter, very widely used in commercial animal breeding, apparently without any higher than normal rate of abnormalities. The embryos either grow normally, Edwards insisted, or they die: 'There are no intermediates.'

This reply did not reassure the critics. They pointed out that there are variations from one species to another in the nature of the reproductive materials. All the animal studies in the world, they said, could not ensure the safety of the first human IVF children.

This clash of opinions led to a dramatic incident at New York's Columbia Presbyterian Hospital, a teaching hospital of Columbia University. In 1973 John and Doris Del Zio were becoming desperate about their inability to produce a child. They read in the press that Shettles had succeeded in fertilizing an egg outside the body, but he had not attempted to transplant the egg into the womb. They went to Shettles and asked him to take one of Doris Del Zio's eggs, fertilize it, and then attempt the transfer of what would be, if it succeeded, the world's first IVF child. On 12 September 1973, the egg was removed and Shettles went ahead with his attempt to fertilize it with John Del Zio's sperm. Then the Chief of Obstetrics at the Columbia Presbyterian Hospital, where Shettles was working, heard of the experiment, which had not been approved by the hospital's Human Experimentation Review Board. Because of the risk of the birth of, as he put it, 'a monstrosity', the Chief terminated the experiment by opening up the flask containing the egg and sperm, thus destroying the culture inside.

The Del Zios sued the Chief of Obstetrics, the university, and the hospital for $1,500,000 for wrongful deprivation of property, and psychological harm. It took so long for the case to be heard that Louise Brown was actually born while the trial was underway. Despite this evidence of the possibility of IVF succeeding, the jury rejected the suit for wrongful deprivation of property, and awarded the Del Zios the more modest sum of $50,003 for psychological harm. (The odd three dollars represented one dollar from each of the three defendents for the husband!)

Fortunately, the first human IVF child is, as far as can be seen, completely normal. So have been virtually all the other IVF babies so far born. (One was born with a heart defect, which was successfully operated on; it is not thought that the defect had any relation to IVF.)

Thus concern over the normality of IVF children has eased, and the extreme statements of Watson, Ramsey, Kass, and the National Research Council Study now appear to have been unduly alarmist. Nevertheless the issue is not quite settled, for two reasons. The first is that the number of IVF children—under 200 at the time of writing—is still too small for anyone to be entirely confident that the rate of abnormal children is no higher than with the usual method of reproduction. This is because the usual rate of abnormalities is low enough for quite a large sample to be—by chance—normal even if IVF in fact produced, say, twice as many abnormalities as ordinary reproduction. Dr Michael Thomas, Chairman of the British Medical Association's Central Ethical Committee, has said: 'We should need about 3,000 test-tube babies before we could be sure the risk isn't there.' Dr J. Schlesselman, writing in the *American Journal of Obstetrics and Gynecology*, has calculated that to have a 90 per cent chance of detecting a doubling of chromosomal abnormalities among IVF children, we would need a sample of more than 2,000 births. Samples of these sizes are still a year or two away.

The second reason that the issue is not settled is that some people have suggested that even though the first IVF babies appear completely normal, we shall not know that they are normal in every respect until we have been able to assess their mental and psychological development up to maturity. With Louise Brown only five years old, this will necessarily take another ten or fifteen years.

While it is true that absolute, cast-iron proof of the physical and mental normality of IVF must await later testing, we do not regard this as a sufficient ground for opposing IVF. The evidence in favour of normal development is already quite strong, and becoming stronger all the time. The argument from the lack of absolute proof is only an argument for careful monitoring of the situation. Moreover, if IVF produced abnormalities, we would expect them to be gross ones, either obvious at birth or in infancy (which has not been the case) or resulting in spontaneous abortion or a failure to implant (which may well be happening).

So the danger that IVF causes some tangible physical or mental damage to the children it produces now appears slight, and in a relatively short time it may well be shown to be non-existent. There have also been, however, suggestions of psychological damage of a different kind. Writing in *The Advocate*, a Melbourne Catholic newspaper, Father Lawrence Fitzgerald referred to 'the distinct possibility of psychological damage to the child' and elaborated as follows:

With all the publicity that has surrounded the *in vitro* births, it is hard to believe that these children will not be ragged at school with: 'Yah! Yah! Yah! You're only an IVF kid!' They may be persuaded that they are odd, in some way; and certainly, that mum and dad were. Or conversely, they could become complete egoists, knowing that, in their generation, they stand apart from the rest of mankind.

The Catholic bishops of Victoria took a similar line in their submission to the Victorian Government Committee on IVF. Referring to 'the long-term relationship between the parents and the child', the bishops asked: 'How can anyone say *a priori*, without extended research at least with non-human primates, that it will make no difference to an IVF child that it was so atypically conceived?' The bishops then urged that 'the Law cannot tacitly acquiesce in a program which would proceed while such a possibility remains unresolved'.

We confess to some puzzlement at the arguments put by the Victorian bishops. One source of this puzzlement is the suggestion that research with non-human primates might enable us to resolve the question of whether 'it will make no difference to an IVF child that it was so atypically conceived'. How exactly do the bishops expect the researchers to convey to the rhesus monkeys, chimpanzees, or gorillas that they were conceived by IVF? Unless this can be conveyed, however, we fail to see how research on non-human primates could have any relevance to the psychological effect, on a human IVF child, of knowing how it was conceived.

There is a more serious ground for our puzzlement. We find it strange that these vague prospects of possible psychological difficulties should be regarded by spokesmen of the Roman Catholic Church as a sufficient ground for opposing IVF. We have to remember that the objection is supposed to apply to the simple case—in which IVF is the only possibility for conception left to a couple otherwise condemned to childlessness. So the argument amounts to this: that because there are some doubts as to the consequences for the parties, the prospective parents should refrain from conceiving at all. But this is not an argument that the Catholic Church is prepared to make at all general. If a young couple told their priest that they wished to avoid conception because they did not feel mature enough to raise a child, he would remind them that marriage was ordained by God, and one of its purposes is the production of children. He would recommend prayer and offer guidance, but would forbid artificial contraception. Or if a woman with a serious hereditary disease told her priest that she wanted to be sterilized to avoid imposing a life of suffering on the child she would bear, he would again forbid it. In no other case does the Catholic Church espouse the view that if pregnancy represents a risk to the child of that pregnancy, then measures guaranteed to avoid the pregnancy should be taken. In the cases imagined above the priest may very well advise the judicious use of the rhythm method, but he would certainly not tell the people concerned that they must follow a course of action which will guarantee that they would not become parents. For infertile couples, however, this is precisely what the bishops' 'no' to IVF comes to.

We can only assume that the reason the bishops judge the two situations so differently is that they have already decided that artificial contraception and artificial fertilization are both intrinsically wrong. This decision must be based on other grounds, presumably on some natural law doctrine of the type we criticized earlier in this chapter. Whatever the grounds, they cannot be simply the risk of psychological damage to offspring: if they were, they would apply in both cases, sanctioning or even requiring contraception in the one case just as firmly as they prohibit IVF in the other.

As for the points made by Fr. Fitzgerald, we have to concede that the publicity associated with being the first IVF baby in the world, or in Australia, or America, may have some effect on the lives of Louise Brown, Candice Reed, and Elizabeth Carr. We very much doubt that this problem of excessive publicity would be anything like as great as it is for children of the British Royal Family (and the danger of psychological damage to royal children has not yet been put forward as an argument for republicanism). We imagine sensible parents will be able to counteract any ill effects from excessive publicity; but even if this were not the case, stopping IVF now would not help to prevent whatever damage had been done to these early IVF children. Indeed stopping IVF now would make matters worse for them, for it would mean that they remained permanent curiosities, the only children ever conceived outside the body. If IVF becomes more and more routine, on the other hand, these early IVF children will come to be less and less unusual. They will be no different from all the other IVF children, apart from the historical significance of the fact that they were the first.

We would not expect the later IVF children to face any special problems. With no publicity over their births, their schoolmates will not know that they are IVF children, unless they choose to tell them. If they do tell them, they might occasionally be teased about it, but is this really a reason for not conceiving them? Would anyone—let alone a Roman Catholic priest—think that because of the danger of their children being teased, people with surnames like 'Smellie' should not reproduce? Nor do we see any grounds for concern over IVF children becoming egoists, especially once their manner of conception becomes routine.

Of course none of this is the hard factual data that the bishops and other critics demand as a condition of accepting IVF. They think the burden of proof is on supporters of IVF to show that their speculations about its possible psychological effects are groundless. But we disagree. If the mere possibility of psychological maladjustments were enough to stop people from having children, then nobody would ever have children. There is no reason why couples who can have children only with the aid of IVF should be singled out and prevented from having families. It would be unacceptable to say to an intending parent that because she was too young, too poor, insufficiently educated, emotionally unstable, a potential child-basher, a drug addict, an alcoholic, or even merely single, that she should be prevented from having children. On the contrary, if they know where to seek it, such people will be given information on the wide range of publicly-funded support services available. Where IVF exists with the aid of public funds, some degree of care may reasonably be demanded. But a consideration of the unfortunate circumstances into which ordinary children can be born vividly illustrates the unreasonably high standards IVF is being asked to meet. There is no evidence to justify these fears. And even if (as we think, improbably) an IVF child did (because of its conception in a dish) suffer psychological hardship, that would hardly make it unique among the human race.

Rupturing the conjugal act

The Church has . . . rejected the . . . attitude which would pretend to separate, in generation, the biological activity in the personal relation of the married couple . . . Never is it permitted to separate these various aspects to the positive exclusion either of the procreative intention or of the conjugal relationship.

So said Pope Paul VI in *Humanae Vitae*. The main intent of the encyclical was to rule out artificial contraception, but the thrust of the argument clearly excludes IVF as well. Paul VI was merely continuing a line of thought expressed previously—and more vividly—by Pius XII:

To reduce the shared life of a married couple and the act of married love to a mere organic activity for transmitting semen would be like turning the domestic home, the sanctuary of the family, into a biological laboratory.

The Victorian Catholic bishops quoted these words in their submission to the Victorian Government Committee inquiring into IVF, and asserted that some non-Catholic bioethicists shared the objection to a process which 'technologizes' a relationship which should be intensely personal. The bishops went on to express their misgivings about any process which separates baby-making from love-making, and to hint at the possibility of IVF damaging the relationship between husband and wife.

It is not up to us to tell Roman Catholic popes or bishops what to think about sexual relations in marriage. Obviously their views on the importance of not separating love and procreation are not widely accepted in societies like ours, in which most couples use artificial means of contraception to plan their families. Nor do the bishops show any awareness of the views of the social workers and counsellors who see infertile couples on a daily basis. Their reports make it plain that childlessness, not IVF, is the great threat to marriage relationships. When couples want a child but cannot have one, each partner is likely to blame the other. The resulting stress can be too much for the marriage to bear. If the bishops were serious in their concern about the effect of IVF on relations between husband and wife, why did they fail to investigate this other side of the issue? Why did they not consult those who work most closely with the infertile?

These points apart, we do once again find it odd that the bishops regard this mere possibility of some unspecified harm as sufficient to override the usual stance of the Church, which is in exactly the opposite direction. In normal circumstances, a refusal to have children, by one partner in a marriage, provides the other partner with grounds for seeking annulment. This is because having children is regarded as the prime purpose of marriage. One might almost think, then, that in a marriage that was infertile because the woman has irreparably damaged Fallopian tubes, if one partner refused to use IVF, the other partner would have grounds for annulment.

In an address to the Italian Catholic Union of Midwives in 1951, Pope Pius XII raised this very question—at that time, he was no doubt thinking of artificial insemination rather than IVF, but the point would apply to both techniques. The Pope acknowledged that the partners in a marriage have 'the right to the child, the primary end of marriage', but he denied that a right to 'artificial fecundation' could be derived from this right to the child: 'The matrimonial contract does not give this right, because it has for its object, not the child, but the natural acts which are capable of engendering a new life and are destined to this end.' This strikes us as a deft avoidance of the issue. In the case of a fertile couple it is all very well to say that the right to a child given by the marriage contract is a right to the natural acts capable of engendering a child; but what about when the natural acts are simply not capable of engendering a new life? If having a child is the primary end of marriage, and this end can only be obtained by artificial insemination or IVF, why doesn't a refusal to use such means strike against the primary purpose of the marriage and hence invalidate it? Again, we suspect a misguided conception of natural law to be lurking behind this curious interpretation of the right the Church normally accords to marriage partners to have a child.

Looking at the matter from an independent perspective, the question to ask is this: Given the unfortunate situation of a married couple who would like to have children, but have no prospect of ever having any unless they use IVF, is their relationship likely to be better if they use IVF, or if they do not?

Infertile couples themselves have no doubt of the answer. Lesley Brown worried about the effect her inability to have a child was having on her marriage. Isabel Bainbridge regards her infertility as a major factor in the breakup of her first marriage. A Darwin woman, writing to Carl Wood for help, described her situation:

I gave myself to the end of this year to become pregnant (having tried to have a baby for the past five years), and I decided that if I wasn't, then I had best leave my husband and let him look for a younger, more productive lady to have babies with.

This will be a very sad thing, as Martin and I have everything going for us, but children.

Jan Brennan also worried:

There were many times when I felt that the fact that I could not have children would have a detrimental effect on Len's love for me and I would often wonder to myself if he would continue to love me as much in the future, and whether our relationship, although very strong and deep, would perhaps suffer through the feelings caused by my infertility.

In contrast to this feeling of the damage childlessness might do to their marriage, the Brennans clearly had no anxiety about the fact that their child had been conceived with the assistance of medical technology. At a Monash University conference on IVF, Len Brennan put it this way:

I considered that we had a mechanical breakdown in our reproductive equipment, and a mechanical repair was necessary by the IVF medical team, to enable us to achieve something natural and beautiful and an essential part of life.

Later in the conference a member of the audience asked a panel of speakers whether it would be feasible to have IVF programmes that incorporate bodily love, for instance by recovering the sperm after intercourse. The panel included Carl Wood as well as Len Brennan, and the question was presumably seeking a medical opinion on whether this method of sperm collection would work. Before Carl Wood could answer, however, Len Brennan rose and replied:

If I may I would like to answer that myself. They say there is no bodily love, but Jan and I have always insisted on having a private room and sperm collection is always an intimate and loving thing between Jan and I. It is done together and it is a very tender time. We do it with total awareness, which is probably more than the average couple does. To us it is very important that she [Pippin] is conceived with love.

On this issue, we find the Brennans more convincing than any number of popes and bishops.

Masturbation

At this point we may as well mention, if only for the sake of completeness, an objection that we are quite unable to take seriously. The normal way of obtaining semen for fertilizing the egg is, of course, masturbation. This can be done by the husband alone, or as we have just seen, it can be done with the assistance of the wife. In either case it is still condemned by some religions, including Roman Catholicism and Orthodox Judaism.

In an address to Catholic doctors in 1949 Pope Pius XII said, referring to the use of artificial insemination: 'It is superfluous to mention that the active element can never be obtained legitimately by means of acts against nature.' More recently, in 1975, a 'Declaration of Certain Questions Concerning Sexual Ethics' was promulgated by the Vatican with the approval of Pope Paul VI. This declaration acknowledged criticisms of the traditional Catholic doctrine on masturbation, including the criticism that masturbation is a normal phenomenon of sexual development. Nevertheless, the declaration continued, 'both the magisterium of the Church . . . and the moral sense of the faithful have declared without hesitation that masturbation is an intrinsically and seriously disordered act'.

For those who follow uncritically the decrees of their religious leaders this is, we suppose, the end of the matter—unless they resort, as Father Laurence Fitzgerald has suggested, to a surgical operation which can obtain sperm direct from the testes! For anyone who is prepared to think independently, however, this is surely the height of absurdity. Masturbation is an entirely normal sexual activity. It is also one of the most harmless acts imaginable. To condemn it as a perversion of the natural function of the sexual organs makes about as much sense as condemning the chewing of sugarless gum as a perversion of the natural function of the mouth.

Even if somehow a valid objection could be made against masturbation for the purpose of sexual pleasure—and we do not for a moment believe it can be—this would have no force against an act of masturbation specifically intended to produce a child. Some Roman Catholic theologians have themselves recognized this difference, but their views have had no effect on official Church doctrines. To condemn masturbation as 'self-abuse' is one thing, but why must a moral outlook be so rigid that it continues to apply this condemnation to every instance of masturbation, notwithstanding the fact that some instances of masturbation are now aimed at fulfilling the procreative function of the sexual organs?

Adoption, not creation?

One frequent objection to IVF is that it is wrong to go to so much trouble and expense to create new babies when there are so many other babies in need of parents to look after them. Couples who cannot have children of their own should adopt these babies instead of resorting to IVF.

If the assumption behind this objection is that there are babies in need of adoption within the community in which IVF is available, then the objection is invalid because that assumption is false, at least as far as countries like Britain, Australia, and the United States are concerned. The legalization of abortion, combined with a tendency for single mothers to keep their babies, has meant that there are now many more couples wishing to adopt than there are healthy babies in need of adoption. (To be strictly accurate, especially in its application to the United States, this statement should refer to 'healthy white babies'—a point which raises a difficult issue, to which we shall return.) Couples wishing to adopt in these countries must meet strict criteria. These criteria exclude couples like the Brennans, in which one partner is over thirty-five. If the couple does meet the criteria, there may still be long waiting-lists.

To find out whether couples seeking IVF would be willing to adopt, we included a question on this topic in a questionnaire we gave to couples either undergoing treatment or awaiting treatment with Carl Wood's IVF team. (A full report of the questionnaire results is in Appendix 2.) We found that of 114 patients, or their husbands, who replied, 72 (or 63 per cent) were willing to use adoption as an alternative means of having a family; 34 per cent said they were not willing to adopt, with the remaining 3 per cent not answering. This confirms the claim often made by those working with IVF patients, that the majority are concerned simply to have a child, and would adopt if there were sufficient babies for adoption. Our finding is also in broad agreement with the Harris poll on IVF taken in the United States in 1978, in which women were asked if they would use the 'test-tube baby' method themselves in preference to adoption, if natural reproduction were difficult or impossible for them: 57 per cent preferred adoption, 21 per cent preferred IVF, and the remainder were either indifferent between the two methods, or unsure of their answer.

There are two variants of the argument that adoption is

preferable to IVF which are not based on an erroneous picture of the availability of babies for adoption. One is that while there may be no surplus of babies for adoption within the affluent nations that can afford IVF, the situation is different in poorer countries. In the slums and shanty towns of much of Asia, Africa, and Latin America, the future is very grim for babies who are orphaned, or simply abandoned by parents who cannot afford to feed them. Rather than create new babies, why should not infertile couples in affluent countries adopt these children and provide them with the food, shelter, and loving care that they so badly need? At the same time, such an adoption programme would make a contribution, albeit a tiny one, to easing the population problem that faces many of the poorer countries. IVF, on the other hand, merely makes an addition—if, once again, a tiny one—to the world population problem.

At present, overseas adoption is being carried out on a small scale. It is a possibility for infertile couples, although it is neither easy nor inexpensive. There is a considerable amount of paperwork required from the authorities of both countries involved. There is also often the expense of a plane trip to pick up the child, including a transition period of two or three weeks in which the child gets used to its new parents. The entire procedure may take three years to be completed.

In our questionnaire we asked the IVF patients and their spouses about their willingness to adopt a child from a poor Asian country (Asia being the usual source of overseas adoption for Australian couples). A majority of the couples (55 per cent) were not prepared to do so, but a significant minority (36 per cent) answered affirmatively, with the remaining 9 per cent not answering.

Something must be done to slow down and eventually stop the population explosion. Neither IVF nor overseas adoption, however, is likely to have any significant impact on this huge problem. The numbers are just too small to make any real difference.

On humanitarian grounds, we would support a properly organized programme enabling couples in affluent countries to adopt orphaned or abandoned children from poorer countries. Yet we see a great difference between the proposition that people in wealthy countries should be encouraged to adopt more third-world orphans, and the proposition that infertile couples who could have children by means of IVF should be denied access to IVF treatment so that they will be forced into adopting third-world orphans, if they are to have any children at all. Adopting a child can be difficult under the best of circumstances—that is why couples seeking adoption are so carefully screened. Adopting a child from another country, a child who will always look different from its parents, and different from most other people in the community in which it lives, is more difficult still. We should not push into this difficult situation people who would much rather have a child that is genetically their own. They may resent the fact that they were not allowed the opportunity to take advantage of modern medical techniques that could have achieved this aim, and this resentment may affect their feelings for the child. The most suitable parents for overseas adoption are likely to be drawn from those who freely choose to have this kind of 'international family'. A more vigorous overseas adoption programme may well be a good thing, and in preliminary counselling sessions prospective IVF patients should be invited to consider it; but there are better ways of bringing it about than denying IVF to those who, after careful consideration of the alternatives, decide that they want it.

A similar reply could be made to those who would argue that IVF is undesirable in the United States, because the shortage of babies for adoption does not extend to black babies. Here too—and especially in view of the extent of racial feeling that still exists there—it would be most unfortunate if people were persuaded into adopting across racial lines when they would much rather have a child of their own genetic descent. In addition, there are some black leaders who object to white adoption of black children, on the grounds that these children will then lose their cultural heritage. (This last point applies to overseas adoption too; it is more rarely heard in this situation because the difference between starving and being well fed is so great as to make such talk out of place.)

The second variant of the adoption argument that is not based on any mistake about the facts, is that it is wrong for us to create new babies for childless couples while at the same time—

sometimes in the same hospital—so many unwanted foetuses are being aborted. Margaret Tighe, leader of Right to Life Australia, has made this point:

> It really does seem crazy . . . Here we are killing off all of these children, and I bet those women who want IVF would give anything to have one of those babies that is being killed at the Royal Women's Hospital right now. We are going to extraordinary lengths creating babies, and we are killing so many off.

Whether abortion is the killing of a child, as Margaret Tighe believes, is not the issue here. She is saying that even from the perspective of making the best possible use of our resources, it seems very odd to be both creating babies and preventing babies from being born. Nor can it be denied that there is a connection between abortion and IVF: by contributing to the reduction in the number of babies needing adoption, legal abortion has increased the pressure from infertile couples for something to be done about their situation.

The problem is that the abortion issue is not simply a matter of whether a foetus lives or dies. There is also the freedom—some would say the right—of the pregnant woman to control her own body and her own life. Women who have abortions are not seeking only to avoid having another child to look after. They are also, or in some cases solely, seeking to avoid pregnancy. To prohibit abortion in order to produce more children for adoption would be to force these women to go through pregnancy and childbirth, against their will, for a child they would give up to another couple. Women might well see this as a kind of reproductive slavery. To justify such a restriction on individual liberty, one would need stronger grounds than the value of the resources that would then not have to be spent on IVF.

There may one day be a way of avoiding the killing of foetal human beings without restricting the freedom of women to control their bodies; but that day is still some time ahead. We discuss this prospect in Chapter 5.

Finally, so far as adoption is concerned, we should make it clear that in denying that adoption provides a sufficient reason for not going ahead with IVF, we have not claimed that couples have a right to have their own genetic children. There probably are many couples who would prefer their children to be 'blood relations' but we do not think that leaving this specific preference unsatisfied causes anything like the distress caused by childlessness itself. As we have seen, most couples seeking IVF would adopt if they could. They want a child and do not mind if it is not the child of their own bodies. We have said that the desire to rear their genetic children may make couples seeking IVF less suitable as adoptive parents, and for this reason we have suggested that they should not be pressured into adoption, especially not overseas or interracial adoption. This suggestion is based on concern for the best interests of the adopted child, and not on a belief that desires for genetic parenthood must be satisfied.

Is it worth the cost?

Despite all the worries that have been expressed about IVF being a step towards Brave New World, and an unnatural intrusion of technology into the act of procreation, the most challenging objection to the simple case of IVF is, in our view, something much more mundane: money.

There is little point in discussing the cost of the research that was required to bring IVF to its present stage of development. Money spent on medical research is always something of a gamble. Quite apart from the successful treatment of infertility that IVF research made possible, it has extended our basic knowledge of reproduction. This could make new modes of contraception possible. It has even been suggested that IVF may make possible new directions in cancer research. These hopes may all come to nothing; but in any case, stopping IVF tomorrow will not recoup what was spent on this basic research.

The cost of the treatment for each patient is another matter. This is a continuing cost, and we must decide if it is justified. As we saw in the preceding chapter, the cost of each egg collection, fertilization, and subsequent transfer of the embryo to the womb, is between $A2,000 and $A4,000. With a success rate for this procedure of no more than 25 per cent, the cost per child produced is in the range of $A10,000 to $A20,000. Is this cost justified?

In the paper he presented to the Ethics Advisory Board inquiry into IVF, Leon Kass argued that it is not:

A conservative estimate might place the cost of a successful pregnancy to be between five and ten thousand dollars. If we use the conservative figure of 500,000 for estimating the number of infertile women with blocked oviducts in the United States whose *only* hope of having children lies in *in vitro* fertilization, we reach a conservative estimated cost of 2.5 to 5 billion dollars. Should technical improvement someday lower the costs to $1,000 per baby, the estimated cost would still be half-a-billion dollars. Is it really even fiscally wise for the Federal Government to start down this road? . . . Much as I sympathize with the plight of infertile couples, I do not believe that they are entitled to the provision of a child at the public expense, especially now, especially at this cost, especially by a procedure that also involves so many moral difficulties.

One reply to those who object to providing infertile couples with children at the public expense, is to say that IVF should be permitted, but only if those couples seeking it are prepared to pay the full cost of treatment. This is in fact the most common situation in America, with the Norfolk clinic charging its patients the full cost, and very few of them being able to obtain coverage from their health insurance. In Australia, on the other hand, we have seen that patients pay at most a third of the full cost, the remainder coming from government-subsidized health insurance funds. In Britain, Edwards and Steptoe's private clinic operates side by side with other centres working within the entirely free National Health Service.

Can one object to the cost of the treatment if it is all borne by the patient? To do so seems excessively paternalistic, for if the couple think that the chance of having a baby is worth the cost—and many obviously do—how can anyone tell them that their decision is unwise? If people are allowed to spend £12,000 on a luxury car, why not on a baby? The problem is that for this argument to work, the couple must really be paying the full cost. If medical students are educated at the public expense, as they are in Britain and Australia, then there is still a hidden subsidy from the taxpayer. Worse still, since the supply of doctors cannot respond quickly to demand, private payment for IVF might divert people with scarce medical skills from other areas where, arguably, they are needed more.

Thus private payment for IVF meets only part of the objections on grounds of cost. In addition, we have to ask if we want to see a situation in which the wealthy infertile are able to have babies, while the poor infertile are not. We might be ready to accept that money makes the difference when it comes to medical treatment that is genuinely optional, like having one's nose straightened; but most people feel differently about medical treatment for some more basic disability. We share this attitude. Whether on grounds of fairness or simply because it is a way of reducing avoidable suffering, we believe that the State should see that all its citizens, irrespective of their means, are provided with basic medical care. But is IVF included within our understanding of basic medical care?

Some critics, Leon Kass among them, have claimed that infertility is not a disease, because the infertile person is as healthy as anyone else—there is no threat to life, nor is there any physical pain or discomfort. Moreover even if infertility were a disease, says Kass, IVF would not be a treatment for it, since IVF—unlike tubal surgery—does not change the underlying condition. It produces a baby, but leaves the woman with blocked tubes as infertile as ever.

Jan Brennan would obviously not agree: 'I am just someone with a disability, a handicap', she has said. 'Obviously there is nothing externally wrong, but it is a disablement.' This is surely correct. There is something physically wrong with a women who has blocked tubes, just as there is something wrong with a person who has lost the use of one hand. Neither condition may be a threat to life, nor a cause of physical pain or discomfort, but both prevent the disabled person from doing one or more things that normal people can do. As for IVF not curing the disability, spectacles do not cure short-sightedness, nor does insulin cure diabetes; yet both are recognized treatments.

So the question is not whether infertility is a medical disability, but how severe a disability it is, and what priority we should give to its treatment, in the light of all the other demands on our medical resources.

In discussing this question, it will be useful to distinguish two possible perspectives from which it may be asked. On the one hand one could ask, 'If we were to distribute in a perfectly rational manner all the resources we now spend on medicine, would we still be allocating resources to test-tube-baby research?'

Alternatively one could ask, 'Given the present overall distribution of medical resources, is there anything particularly inappropriate about the amount we are spending on test-tube-baby research?'

The first of these perspectives attempts to measure the amount we spend on test-tube babies against some ideal standard; the second measures it against the standard of our current pattern of expenditure. Obviously these are very different standards. In an ideal world, each dollar of medical expenditure would be used to maximum effect to eliminate illness and disability wherever it occurs. Thus we would not have a situation in which millions of children die from malnutrition (and from the diseases that afflict the malnourished because they are too weak to resist) while major hospitals develop coronary care units that are marvels of technology but of uncertain value in saving lives. There can be little doubt that more lives would be saved by providing adequate food and a very basic level of health care for those who need it than by providing the latest electronic equipment for heart-attack victims. This kind of redistribution, however, would require the wealthy nations to share more equally with the poorer nations, and this is something that the wealthy nations have so far been unwilling to do.

Even if we limit our attention to a single nation such as Australia, similar irrationalities in the use of medical resources are not hard to find. Once again, the large sums spent on the most sophisticated forms of intensive care would be difficult to justify when compared with the relatively small amounts required to make real inroads into infant mortality, blindness, and infectious disease among Aborigines.

We may lament this situation; we may—we should—try to change it; but we would be unrealistic if we did not acknowledge that there are powerful institutional barriers to an ideally rational ordering of medical expenditure. Those in leading positions in politics, the media, the civil service, and the medical establish-ment can be expected to have built-in bias towards more resources for the kind of conditions from which they, their families, and their friends are likely to suffer, and these conditions include heart attacks but not malnutrition-related diseases. Moreover, doctors and medical researchers themselves are naturally attracted towards those areas of research and treatment that present the most interesting challenges to their intellect and skill. These are not necessarily the areas that offer the greatest benefits to patients per dollar spent.

Hence to assess spending on IVF against an ideally rational scale of priorities is to apply a standard so exacting that it would condemn a good deal of widely accepted medical expenditure. If we are considering the ethics of IVF in particular, rather than undertaking a general assessment of all medical expenditure, this is an unduly stringent standard to apply.

Measured against the standard of our current expenditure, IVF does not look bad. As we saw in the previous chapter, IVF costs less than microsurgery to repair damaged tubes. At present, the slightly lower success rate per laparoscopy of IVF means that it may be a slightly less cost-effective way of overcoming infertility, but the difference is not great and could easily tilt the other way if IVF success rates continue to improve. Defenders of IVF might therefore ask Leon Kass whether his doubts about a couple's right to a child at public expense should not also lead to the rejection of tubal surgery, unless the full costs are met privately.

Some other comparisons may be relevant. One treatment that obviously is life-saving is dialysis for people whose kidneys are not working. The treatment of one person on renal dialysis for one year costs, in Australia, $A27,000. At the other end of the scale of need, the official Australian list of fees that may be recovered from medical benefit funds includes such items as the augmentation of a breast, for 'significant breast asymmetry' or following breast removal. The medical fee that may be claimed for this is $A315, in addition to around $A60 for the anaesthetic, and hospital charges. Hair transplantation can also be claimed, if the loss of hair is not normal male baldness, at a fee of $A200, plus anaesthetist's and hospital charges.

In our view, treatment for IVF is a lower priority than kidney dialysis, but *at least* as high a priority as cosmetic surgery for breast augmentation or a hair transplant. We would also put IVF on a similar footing to psychiatric services aimed at overcoming stress or anxiety, which may also be claimed on health funds. We base this view on the fact that infertility is itself a cause of severe anxiety and depression for the infertile couple. The reports of social workers and counsellors of the infertile show that infertility can be a major life crisis, causing severe stress to the marriage, isolation from other friendships (often becaue of the pain of seeing other couples with their children), feelings of helplessness at the inability to fulfil a basic life goal, and a sense of guilt and unworthiness at not providing one's spouse with a child, and one's parents with grandchildren.

The infertile agree. Isabel Bainbridge, who before trying IVF had two major operations to repair her damaged Fallopian tubes, which resulted only in two ectopic pregnancies, has said:

People who complain about the cost of infertility research and the IVF program should examine the cost to the community of the long-term unhappiness associated with infertility. The cost cannot be counted financially. In the long-term the most cost-effective treatments will be reasonably safe and quick and cheap to perform while leaving minimal physical damage to the patient. IVF and artificial insemination both seem to meet these requirements. Yet governments still prefer to spend public money by funding the sometimes more expensive, more dangerous, less successful major operations as treatments for infertility.

Barbara Menning, an infertile American woman who also had unsuccessful surgery and other invasive medical treatments, founded a group called Resolve, to offer advocacy and support for the infertile. She believes that those who are fertile cannot really understand what the infertile suffer:

At the Ethics Advisory Board hearings, it was amazing how many 'right to lifers' and other witnesses stood up and gave among their credentials the number of children they had borne, as if to add credibility to their testimony. In my opinion, and in the opinion of other infertile women, the fact that they had achieved their families *disqualified* them from any understanding of the pain of childlessness.

Consistently with the views of Isabel Bainbridge and Barbara Menning, the IVF patients responding to our questionnaire overwhelmingly believed that all the costs of their treatment should be rebateable under the national health insurance scheme, as is the case with other medical expenses: 93 per cent took this view; only 6 per cent disagreed. We then asked the patients and their spouses if they would be able to afford to remain on the IVF programme if they were no longer able to claim some of their expenses on health insurance: 7 per cent said that they would not be able to afford IVF at all, while another 12 per cent said they would be able to afford only one attempt; 64 per cent thought they could afford a limited number of treatments, and 14 per cent indicated that 'money is no barrier'.

In our view the top priorities in the provision of health services should be saving lives—as long as the person saved will have a tolerable quality of life—and the relief of serious pain and suffering. Most economically developed nations, of course, do use public funds to see that all members of the community have access to medical services that go well beyond saving lives and relieving serious physical pain. They also allocate public resources to treating other disabilities and to relieving serious mental suffering. IVF falls into these last two categories.

We think it would be absurd for the public purse to pay for a psychiatrist to attempt to treat the depression and anxiety caused by infertility, but not to pay for the treatment of infertility itself. The desire for children is, in many people, something very basic and cannot be overcome without great difficulty, if at all. There are obvious evolutionary reasons why this should be so. We consider that it is quite appropriate for an affluent society to spend public funds on assisting its citizens to satisfy this desire.

The final decision about where money is best spent will depend on the particular circumstances, and is always open to argument. Here we are only considering the general objection that it is wrong to spend community resources on IVF. We do not find that, in general, there is any sound reason why a reasonably affluent society should not spend some of its resources on IVF. There must, of course, be a limit to how much is spent. Spending in this area should not be allowed to cut into spending in other areas of greater priority. Government expenditure, however, is to some extent flexible, and it is a mistake to assume that a million dollars spent on IVF means a million dollars less spent on kidney dialysis. Perhaps governments need to spend more on health as a whole.

The simple case: conclusions

Despite the fact that the 'simple case' of IVF was tailored to avoid as many objections as possible, it has had to meet several challenges. Any use of IVF at all has been said to be wrong because it is unnatural, because it is a step down the slippery slope toward a society like Brave New World, because it might produce abnormal children, because it separates baby-making from love-making, because adoption is preferable, and, finally, because it is not worth the cost.

We have now examined all these objections. Some, like the charge of unnaturalness, the slippery slope objection, and the rupturing of sex and procreation, we were able to dismiss in what we believe to be a conclusive manner. In considering the justifiability of IVF in the simple case, we do not think these objections need be given any weight at all. One other objection—the risk of abnormal children—cannot yet be dismissed conclusively, but it is beginning to look as if it will be possible to do so in another year or two. The desirability of increasing overseas adoption does carry some weight against the too-ready use of IVF, but its impact should not extend beyond counselling—it is not a good reason for preventing the use of IVF where overseas adoption is impractical or the couple are adamant in their preference for IVF.

The final question, that of cost, proved difficult to discuss in the abstract. When we looked at other medical services for which some kind of public subsidy is commonly available in developed nations, it did not seem unreasonable for IVF to be covered in a similar manner. Nevertheless, unless the cost of IVF can be sharply reduced, it will always be possible to argue that there are better ways of using our medical resources. This is a decision that each society must make in the light of what its medical needs are and what it can afford to provide. The cost of IVF is therefore not an insuperable objection to all uses of IVF, but in certain times and places it may provide a reason for not offering this relatively expensive form of infertility treatment.

3 IVF: BEYOND THE SIMPLE CASE

IVF for whom?

If there is no sound reason to condemn the use of IVF in the simple case, what extensions beyond the simple case are justifiable? To probe this question we shall query each of the restrictions that were present in the simple case. The first of these limited IVF to a married couple. Should this treatment be restricted to married couples? Or should it also be available to unmarried couples, or to single women?

In discussing whether IVF should be provided from public funds, we saw that in many ways IVF is analogous to other forms of medical treatment. It is now widely accepted that medical treatment should be available to all those in need of it, irrespective of social class, religion, life-style, or moral character. The need for IVF can be established by the strength of the desire for children. Anyone prepared to go through the daunting experience of fertility tests, multiple examinations, counselling, and laparoscopy, as required for IVF, will undoubtedly have a strong desire for a child. The burden of proof would therefore seem to be on those who believe that IVF should be allocated on some basis other than the need of the patient.

Presumably the argument for restricting IVF to married couples is that the children should have a good home. But different people have different views as to what constitutes a good home. Anyone seeking IVF, whether married or not, would be doing it with the child in mind, and with every intention of furnishing it with a good home. Whatever anyone else thought of such people's sexual mores, they would not be going through IVF for fun.

We know of no empirical research which demonstrates that

married couples provide children with a better home environment than, for instance, unmarried couples in a long-standing relationship. In any case, even if such generalizations were supported by evidence, they could never show that *particular* unmarried people would not provide children with a good home. That judgement can only be made on the basis of all the facts of the particular case. We are not opposed to people being rejected for IVF treatment if there are substantial reasons for believing that they would not provide the child with a good home; but we are opposed to a prohibition against a whole class of people, which would not allow each case to be judged on its merits.

Modern societies do not seek to prevent any fertile people, whatever their marital status or private sexual preference, from reproducing. Why then should they single out the infertile for special control over reproduction? The only plausible argument for doing so is that since society has provided at least some of the funds for the treatment, it has the responsibility for making sure they are used wisely, and not used to create children who will suffer from their poor start in life. We could accept such an argument, as long as the selection procedures were carefully designed to screen out *only* those people who would be likely to give the child a poor start in life. Unless there is some factual basis for the belief that unmarried couples are less likely to provide a good home, a blanket exclusion of the unmarried is nothing more than discrimination against the nonconforming.

The same point applies to the exclusion of single women or lesbian couples. Is it really true that they could not provide a child with a good home? We wonder whether this could possibly be true in all cases. If it cannot be shown always to be true, selection procedures should not exclude these people as a class. They would, of course, require donated sperm, which is also outside the 'simple case'. We shall come to this in the next section.

If the blanket restriction to married couples is insupportable, what about the restriction to infertile couples? Should IVF be available for couples who could have a child by the normal method?

To pose this question is to invite another: why should anyone want to use IVF if they can reproduce normally? There is, however, an answer. If a man carries a serious genetic defect, one way of not passing the defect on is to use AID; that is, for the female partner to be artificially inseminated with sperm provided by a donor. When it is the woman who carries the genetic defect, however, this technique is no use. Until the advent of IVF there was only one way for the woman to have a child without running the risk of passing on the defect. If the defect could be detected during pregnancy, an abortion could be performed and afterwards the woman could try again. Apart from the obvious disadvantage of abortion, this method cannot be applied in the case of genetic defects which are not detectable during pregnancy. With the use of IVF, however, there is another way. Just as donor sperm can be used to replace the genetically defective sperm, so a donor egg could be used to replace the egg of the woman with the genetic defect. IVF with a donor egg is the flip side of AID. Since AID may be used to avoid passing on a genetic defect, it is obviously not restricted to couples in which the male is infertile. Unless we encounter, in the next section, some valid objection to the use of donor eggs we shall have to conclude that IVF should also not be restricted to infertile couples.

Before we leave this topic, we shall report the views of the IVF couples responding to our questionnaire. These were, incidentally, all married couples, in accordance with the selection criteria used by Carl Wood's team. By 62 per cent to 33 per cent, they supported the admission to IVF programmes of infertile couples who are not married but have 'a stable *de facto* relationship'. They clearly rejected, however, the admission of women without a current male partner (19 per cent for, 73 per cent against) and of lesbians or other women not wishing to have a sexual relationship with a man (15 per cent for, 78 per cent against).

Donor sperm

In the simple case, the egg and sperm came from the married couple themselves. Is there any ethical basis for this restriction? We shall first consider the use of donated sperm.

Sperm from a donor, rather than from the husband, has been used in IVF treatments in Melbourne and at some other centres, and pregnancies have resulted. The reason for using donor sperm is usually that in addition to the wife having blocked tubes or some other defect in her reproductive system, the husband has no sperm or not enough to achieve fertilization. Another possible reason would be that the husband carries a genetic defect. The children born as a result of this particular combination of IVF and AID are the genetic descendants of their mothers, but not of the man they will regard as their father.

If IVF and AID are in themselves both ethically acceptable, we cannot see how there could be a valid objection to IVF with donor sperm. There may be circumstances in which the mixing of two harmless practices results in something far from harmless, but what peculiar catalytic effects could this particular combintion have? We know of none.

Any objection to the use of donor sperm in IVF would therefore have to apply to AID as well. So we might deal with the issue simply by pointing out that AID has been widely used for many years, and is not under any threat of being stopped. In the United States it has been estimated that 100,000 AID children had been born by the year 1957, and the total must now be several times that figure, with approximately 20,000 American women reeiving AID each year. In other Western nations AID does not have such a long history of widespread use, but its use has increased dramatically in the past decade. In these circumstances any prohibition of the use of donor sperm in IVF would seem quite inconsistent with the continuing use of AID.

Tempting as this quick way of disposing of the issue may be, it would invite the reply that no matter how widely it is used, opposition to AID does exist. Unless we have shown that this opposition is unwarranted, we risk using the existence of one unethical practice as a justification for starting another. Hence we need to take a brief look at the opposition to AID.

Readers of the previous chapter will not be surprised to learn that Pope Pius XII emphatically rejected AID. This remains the official attitude of the Roman Catholic Church. Non-religious worries about AID have centred on the right of the child to know about his or her origins, and the possibility of incestuous marriage between half-siblings who are, unknown to them, the offspring of the same sperm donor. There is also, in many countries, some uncertainty about the legal status of children conceived through AID; but this situation can be satisfactorily resolved by legislation which declares them to be the legitimate children of the husband who consents to his wife using AID.

Roman Catholic opposition to AID is based on the broad grounds we have already discussed: the severing of procreation from sexual intercourse, and the objection to masturbation. We need not repeat our reasons for dismissing these arguments. The risk of unwitting incest turns out to be so low that it does not amount to a serious worry—according to one calculation, if there were 2,000 AID children born in Britain each year, and each donor had been responsible for five children, an accidental incestuous marriage would be unlikely to occur more than once in fifty to a hundred years. Moreover, nine times out of ten the children of half-siblings would be completely normal.

The major remaining ethical worry about AID is whether the child will or will not be told of his or her origins, and what might happen in each case. AID is much easier to keep secret than adoption, since the mother goes through a normal pregnancy, and the child is likely to show some family resemblance to one parent. On the other hand one can never be sure that the secret will be kept: the father may, in a fit of rage or spite at a child that does not behave as he would like it to, suddenly announce that he is not the child's 'real' father anyway. Or the mother may tell the child the truth as a way of weakening the influence over the child of a husband with whom she has quarrelled. In these strained circumstances such a revelation would come as a psychological shock that some children would find difficult to take. More rarely, the truth might also have to come out if the father should prove to have an inheritable disease, and the child is worried about also having it.

Unsuccessful attempts to keep AID secret could thus cause problems; but even if the secret is kept, the situation is far from ideal. The child is being deceived. The deception may not do any harm, but it could be argued that the child has a right to the truth on an important matter like this. Moreover, can one be sure that the deception does not do harm? Does it not place some strain on close family relationships for the parents to keep the truth from their child?

We are not sure about the answer to the last question, but all in all it would seem much better for AID parents to tell their children as soon as they are capable of understanding. Many AID practitioners have swung round to this view, and are counselling the parents accordingly. This does, however, raise another problem. Children who are told that they were conceived with the sperm of a donor will be curious about their genetic father. Indeed, if the experience of adopted children is anything to go by, some will be more than simply curious. The desire to know about their genetic father may become a dominating force; if left unfulfilled, the resulting gap in their knowledge of their origins could be a major source of unhappiness. On the other hand, many AID practitioners believe that it is essential to preserve the anonymity of the sperm donor. They believe that men will not donate sperm if at some later stage their children will be able to identify them and perhaps even make demands upon them.

There are two possible ways of dealing with this situation. The first is to allow the release to the child only of general, non-identifying data about the characteristics of the donor. This would partially satisfy the child's desire for knowledge, and would not threaten the donor. The other, more radical proposal, is to release to the child at the age of eighteen the identity of the sperm donor. This would, of course, require the consent of the donor before making the donation; but there is now some evidence that this would not bring the abrupt end to donations that some AID practitioners fear. According to a study of AID donors conducted by Robyn Rowland of Deakin University, in Victoria, 61 per cent of donors interviewed were willing to have their identity made known to their AID children who had reached the age of eighteen, and to have provision made for contact with them. This is despite the fact that the law in Victoria still does not recognize AID, and hence a child by AID might be able to claim an inheritance from his or her genetic father. (Reform of this law has been accepted in principle by the Victorian government; like reforms in some United States jurisdictions, the effect will be to make the AID child the legal child of the husband of the mother, as long as the husband has consented to the use of AID.)

If the results of Rowland's research are confirmed elsewhere, the dilemma of 'to tell or not to tell' will have a straightforward solution: tell. Even if the early results are not repeated in other groups of donors the release of non-identifying data would reduce the severity of the problem. In any case, the problem is not so weighty as to override the reasons for using AID. Some parents will handle the situation poorly, and some children will suffer psychologically as a result, but even these children will not suffer to the point at which they would rather not have been born. And that, surely, is the alternative: without AID these children would not have existed at all. If their lives remain well worth living despite the psychological difficulties, and if AID satisfies the deep desire of the couple for a child, then it is difficult to see how AID could be condemned on the grounds of its possible consequences for child or parents.

Now we can return to IVF. We said that any objection to the use of donor sperm in IVF would have to be an objection to AID as well. We have found that AID can give rise to some ethical problems, but that on the whole it is an ethically acceptable procedure. This conclusion can be straightforwardly applied to the use of donor sperm in IVF, if the male partner is infertile or carries a genetic defect. As in AID, parents should be counselled about the desirability of informing their children of all the circumstances of their birth, and records of sperm donors should be kept to allow non-identifying data to be released to the child upon request. Under these conditions, the use of donor sperm does not add any objectionable element to the simple case of IVF.

In the previous section we suggested that single women or lesbian couples might be able to show their ability to provide a child with a good home, and they should then be eligible for IVF. The acceptability of the use of donor sperm removes another possible objection to this extension beyond the simple case.

Donor eggs

What of donor eggs? We have already seen that by using the egg of another woman, a mother could avoid passing on a genetic defect to her child. It could also, of course, be a way of overcoming infertility in a woman who was not ovulating. Both these situations are quite parallel to the use of donor sperm to overcome male infertility or a genetic defect carried by the male. If the use of a donated egg appears more bizarre, that is only because women bearing children who are not the genetic children of their husbands is as old as adultery; women bearing children who are not their own genetic children is something entirely new.

The major difference between the two is that sperm is easily obtained by masturbation, whereas eggs can only be collected by means of laparoscopy, which involves an operation under general anaesthesia. This is not, however, a major problem. Women undergoing IVF are routinely treated with fertility drugs to stimulate them to produce several eggs. Frequently half a dozen or more eggs are produced. Since the fertilization rate is around 90 per cent and no more than three embryos are transferred to the womb, this procedure commonly produces eggs that are surplus to the needs of the woman from whom they were taken. Since women undergoing IVF are well aware of the misery infertility can cause, many of them are very willing to donate these surplus eggs to other infertile women.

The only remaining problem is the technical one of synchronizing the cycles of the donor woman and the woman who will receive the egg, so that the womb of the latter will be in the right condition to receive the egg after it has been fertilized with the sperm of her male partner. This can be achieved by the use of hormones; alternatively, with a large enough group of donors, it might be possible to find one whose cycle coincided naturally. Reliable methods of freezing and thawing embryos would eliminate the need to synchronize the cycles. In any case, Carl Wood's team in Melbourne has succeeded in obtaining .a pregnancy from a donor egg, so the difficulty is obviously soluble.

These differences between the use of donor sperm and donor eggs do not cause any ethical difficulties. Ethically, the use of donor eggs is on a par with the use of donor sperm. Legally, it could be dealt with in the same manner, the child being declared the legitimate child of the woman who receives the egg and bears the child.

Donor embryos

Donor sperm is all right; donor eggs are all right: what if the two are combined? This amounts to the donation of an embryo, although the two donors whose egg and sperm have united to create the embryo may not know each other, nor may they know that between them they have produced a child.

The first successful pregnancy from a donated embryo was reported by Carl Wood's team in 1983. The donor of the egg was a forty-two-year-old patient on the IVF programme. After the usual hormone treatment, five eggs were collected from her, three were fertilized with her husband's semen and transferred to her womb. One of the remaining eggs was donated to another patient on the programme. This patient, the recipient, had a husband who was infertile; moreover, although the patient produced eggs herself, she had had twenty-three attempts at AID without becoming pregnant. She was considered for IVF with donor sperm, but the medical team advised her that laparoscopy was risky because she had suffered from a thrombosis. The patient said she preferred to receive a donated egg than to risk a laparoscopy or give up the chance of pregnancy.

The donated egg was fertilized with sperm from an anonymous donor. The embryo was then transferred to the recipient, who became pregnant. Some ten weeks after the transfer, however, the pregnancy spontaneously aborted. Examination of the aborted foetus showed that it had an abnormal condition known as a trisomy of chromosome 9. Foetuses with this abnormality have not been known to live.

After publishing their report of this pregnancy in the *British Medical Journal*, Wood and his team found themselves under attack from an unusual quarter: Patrick Steptoe and Robert Edwards. In a letter to the *British Medical Journal*, Steptoe and Edwards asked why an egg from a forty-two-year-old donor had been used. Women in this age group, they said, were known to be at risk for producing abnormal foetuses. Why had not a younger donor been used? Steptoe and Edwards disagreed, too, with the medical advice given to the recipient: they did not think her condition made laparoscopy risky. They also asked whether the donor had been offered the option of storing the donated egg for her own use at a later stage. Pointing out that the donor was near the end of her reproductive life, Steptoe and Edwards wondered if the donation was not reducing her own prospects of pregnancy, and if she should have been allowed to donate an embryo under these circumstances. They concluded by saying that the history of the case was 'strongly suspicious of hurried decisions under pressure' and that it illustrated the need for 'firm ethical guidelines' to be set up.

In reply, Alan Trounson, Carl Wood, and John Leeton acknowledged that in an ideal world they would have used an egg from a younger donor; but no such egg was available to them at the time. They said that the recipient had been informed of the age of the donor, and it was her decision to receive it rather than undergo an operation for egg collection. As for the donor, she was given the option of using all her eggs for immediate embryo transfer, using some and storing some, or anonymously donating extra eggs to other women. It was her choice to donate an egg. Their own ethos, they said, had developed under the guidance of two Hospital Ethics Committees as well as a University Committee and the National Health and Medical Research Council. This ethos, they said, differed from that of Steptoe and Edwards in that while the committees laid down general guidelines, the final decisions were made by the patients and the doctors on the basis of fully informed consent:

We do not dictate to patients who should or should not attempt to conceive . . . Many couples would not wish to receive an egg from a 42-year-old woman, but we reserve the right to assist in the donation, should the fully informed donor and recipient couples desire this.

This public row between the world's two leading IVF groups should not obscure the fact that Steptoe and Edwards were not objecting to embryo donation in itself, but rather to the particular case in which it was used by the Melbourne team. Nor does the public appear to reject embryo donation, although it approves of it by a much narrower margin than it approves of IVF in the simple case. The poll taken in Australia in July 1982 and in Britain in September 1982 included this question:

It's been suggested that fertilized eggs could, with the permission of the husband and wife, be given to another married couple who can't have children, so they can have a child. Do you approve or disapprove of that?

In Australia, 45 per cent approved, 30 per cent disapproved and 25 per cent had no opinion or needed to know more. In Britain 41 per cent approved and 36 per cent disapproved.

Embryo donation could become more widespread by making use of a method much simpler than IVF. In July 1983 Dr John Buster, of the Harbour–UCLA Medical Center in Torrance, California, reported that his team had achieved two pregnancies by transferring fertilized eggs from donor women to infertile women. Surgery was not required because the fertilized eggs were removed through the vagina. This method, known as intra-uterine transfer, should be easier and cheaper than creating embryos outside the womb by *in vitro* fertilization. It could even be done on an out-patient basis, like AID. Pregnancy could be achieved by normal sexual intercourse or, if only an egg rather than an embryo were needed—in other words, if the husband was fertile—the donor could be artificially inseminated with the husband's sperm. In fact Carl Wood's team has recently reported—in January 1984—the first successful birth from a donated embryo.

Whether the technique used is an intra-uterine transfer or IVF, if the husband's sperm cannot be used, the child will not be genetically related to either of its parents. The situation will be very much like that of an adopted child—so much so that Carl Wood's team refers to embryo donation as 'pre-natal adoption'. In some respects embryo donation is to be preferred to adoption, for the genetic mother did not have to bear the child, and thus parting with it would, presumably, be that much easier; what is more, the adopting parents would have the experience of pregnancy and childbirth, and consequently may feel that much closer to the child in its first few weeks. As Roger Short puts it: 'You don't adopt a 10 year old child, you try and adopt a newborn baby. Even better than adopting a newborn baby is to adopt a fertilized egg.'

Is this enough to show that the use of the donor embryo is at least as acceptable as adoption? Not quite. One reason—perhaps the major reason—why we approve of adoption is that it is in the best interests of an existing child. Adoption is desirable when it is the best way of coping with the unfortunate situation of a child without a parent who is willing or able to care for it. Embryo donation is the deliberate creation of an individual who would not otherwise have existed. It is not so much like existing adoption programmes, as like a programme of creating babies so that they can be adopted by infertile couples.

The strongest objection to embryo donation is that the possible adverse psychological effects of learning that one's father or mother is not one's genetic parent would have much greater impact when this applies to both parents. In *this* respect, however, the problem is not greater than adoption. We have some experience of the difficulties suffered by adopted children. Like the difficulties of AID, they should not be minimized, but they should also not be exaggerated. They can be alleviated by keeping records so that the children can later make contact with—or at least have some knowledge of—their genetic parents. In any case, these difficulties do not render the lives of the children involved so miserable that anyone could reasonably judge it better that the child had never been born. So as with AID, it seems impossible to disapprove of embryo donation because of its effect on the children created by it. Its effect on the infertile couple is, of course, beneficial, for it makes it possible for them to have their much-desired child. Embryo donation is thus an acceptable extension of IVF.

Love or money?

The transfer of sperm in AID is already a routine procedure. Since there are no insuperable difficulties, neither medical nor ethical, in the transfer of eggs and embryos, we expect that in the near future this too will become routine. The question is, what sort of system should we establish for the transfer of these human reproductive materials?

The basic alternatives are a system of voluntary donation, like the system of blood donation in Britain and Australia, or a free-market system, like the system for the private sale of blood which provides some of the blood used for medical purposes in the United States. In between these two extremes of pure altruism and pure commerce lie a range of other possibilities. A system of voluntary donation could be modified by the payment of compensation for the time and trouble of the donor. A commercial system might be regulated so that instead of the price being set by supply and demand, the state fixes a price at what it considers a reasonable level.

The market systems and the system of pure voluntary donation are clear enough, but it may be helpful to illustrate the idea of voluntary donation plus compensation. This is, in fact, the system by which, in several countries, sperm is obtained for AID. A sperm donor in Australia is asked for a minimum of five donations, before each of which he will have had to abstain from sexual intercourse or masturbation for three days. The abstinence is necessary to maximize the sperm count. Five donations are necessary in order to provide enough genetic material to make a single conception probable. Sperm banks prefer fifteen donations from each donor. This is to ensure that if a husband and wife seeking AID wish to have more than one child, those children really will be siblings rather than half siblings. They will have the same genetic mother, and come from the sperm of the same donor. Before donating, each donor has to undergo a rigorous questionnaire concerning his own and his family's medical history. Then there is the commitment of time. For each block of five donations the donor receives $A50, which represents compensation for fifteen days abstinence, perhaps five hours at the sperm bank producing the material, however many hours travel time, and of course travel costs. And while the operation by which the genetic material is obtained is not exactly painful, it is an operation that he will not have performed for three days— enough time for many men to feel a noticeable degree of frustration. Few sperm donors would go into it for the money. But they might well appreciate the compensation for their inconvenience. This should illustrate just why a sperm donor would see that $A50 as compensation rather than payment for his genetic material.

The issue, then, is whether a market system is preferable to a voluntary donation system, either in its pure form or modified to allow for compensation for inconvenience. Let us look first at a roughly parallel debate, that concerning blood donation. In favour of the voluntary system it has been argued that it delivers at least as much blood; that the blood is of superior quality (since voluntary donors will have no incentive for misleading others about their medical history, for example whether they have had hepatitis); that it leads to more efficient use of blood, since commercial blood bank systems waste blood and have an incentive to promote excessive use of their product; and that it provides people with an opportunity to express a healthy altruism towards their fellow citizens.

Against this it has been argued that sometimes a voluntary system cannot deliver enough, and that to prohibit the sale of blood is to limit the freedom of those who wish to engage in that kind of economic activity—or as the American philosopher Robert Nozick has put it, to interfere with 'capitalist acts between consenting adults'. Claims of wastage in the commercial system have been challenged, and some commercial blood banks have been able to avoid a high rate of hepatitis by careful selection of their suppliers.

Arguments of a different order are added to the debate on both sides. It has been argued against the voluntary system that we should not recklessly use up the 'scarce resources of altruistic motivation', and for the voluntary system that altruism is a renewable resource, which rather than disappearing through over-use, will atrophy if not called upon. These opposing views rest upon different views of human nature. Perhaps each of us can, by introspection, cast some light on the issue of the exhaustibility or renewability of altruism, but a decisive means of determining the issues does not exist.

Let us now apply these considerations to the different question of drawing up the rules for a new institution, for example, for egg donation. And let us begin with the more intractable problem. Either human altruism will prove sufficient to meet the demand or it will not. And either we will set up a voluntary system or we will set up a commercial system. If we are starting out in a new area, with which system should we begin?

Suppose we set up a voluntary system, in the hope that human altruism will prove sufficient, but we have been too generous in our judgement of our fellow humans. They are not as altruistic as we imagined them to be. The system does not work—too few donations are forthcoming. This would rapidly be discovered, and it would be necessary to institute a system of payments. Except in the short term, no harm would have been done by our error of judgement.

What if we made the opposite error, setting up a commercial system because we had judged our fellow humans too harshly? Obviously we could be missing out on any advantages that might flow from making a call on human altruism that it is, unknown to us, well able to sustain. What might those advantages be?

Institutionalizing, in a new area, the habit of acting altruistically, can have good effects. As Richard Titmuss argued in *The Gift Relationship*, it can strengthen the bonds between strangers by providing opportunities for people to relate unselfishly to their fellow citizens. An institution based on altruism thus has a sort of spill-over effect on the rest of social life, reducing the dominance of the market-place—where we attempt to profit from our dealings with our fellow citizens—and bringing the community together. Once we have set up a commercial system, unfortunately, we shall have no way of learning our error, and we shall never know that these advantages were within our reach.

Should we then opt for the voluntary system and hope that human altruism will be sufficient to sustain it? We have seen that even if we are wrong, we stand to lose much less if we opt first for the voluntary system, than if we start with a commercial system. So we can conclude that when establishing such institutions, it is best to try a voluntary system first.

To this abstract argument in favour of setting up a voluntary system, we can add the practical point that in this specific area there is every reason to expect an adequate supply of eggs from voluntary donations. As long as there are patients in IVF programmes producing surplus eggs, a woman donating an egg can do so without inconvenience and without harming her own chances of becoming pregnant. We would expect most of these women to be very willing to donate surplus eggs to other infertile women. There would be no need to offer a monetary incentive.

To check this belief, in our survey of IVF couples we asked if they thought it all right for excess eggs or embryos to be made available for donation, either immediately or after freezing. They approved of donation by margins of around 75 per cent to 15 per cent, with 10 per cent undecided (the exact figures varied slightly according to whether the question related to eggs or embryos, and to immediate donation or donation after freezing). We also asked if they thought an IVF couple should be able to sell their embryos. Of 112 people who answered the question, 111 thought that selling should not be permitted.

Should IVF techniques change at some future date, so that fertility drugs are no longer used and surplus eggs are no longer produced, the adequacy of a voluntary system would come under greater strain. To ask a woman to undergo a laparoscopy purely in order to donate an egg to someone else is asking much more than we ask of a blood donor. There may be enough women who would do it; we cannot tell. In any case, at present fertility drugs and surplus eggs are a standard part of IVF techniques, and there is no reason to expect this to change.

There is also another method of obtaining donated eggs. Women undergoing tubal sterilization can donate an egg without any additional inconvenient medical procedure. If they are willing to have a hormone administered to stimulate the production of several eggs, more eggs can be obtained without additional risk. In Britain, eggs used for research purposes have already been obtained from such voluntary donations.

The weight of argument, both abstract and practical, is clearly in favour of setting up a voluntary system for egg donation. As long as IVF patients produce surplus eggs, it could be a pure voluntary system, for the patients do not suffer any inconvenience as a result of making the donation. Sperm donors, on the other hand, do have to give up their time to make the donations, and they have to put up with some inconvenience (how much depends on their sexual habits). A modified voluntary system, like that described earlier, is appropriate here. The important point is that any financial compensation offered should be too small to be the prime motivation for the donation. Quite apart from the desirability of fostering altruism, what has to be avoided is any possibility of the money inducing the donor to conceal details of his family history which would make his sperm less likely to be accepted.

Embryo donation does not need to be considered separately from the donation of the eggs and sperm. We assume that where an embryo is needed by a couple, the egg and sperm will be procured separately through the programme set up for egg donation and sperm donation.

Embryo wastage

In the simple case, no more eggs are to be fertilized than the woman is prepared to have transferred to her womb. The idea behind this requirement is, of course, that no embryos are left over to be frozen, donated to other women, dissected for research purposes, experimented upon, or just tipped down the sink. The most vexed of all the ethical issues associated with IVF—the debate over the moral status of the embryo—is thus avoided. The strongest political opposition to IVF has come from right-to-life organizations, who insist that from the moment of conception there is a human being with as much of a right to life as any other human being. When IVF is carried out in accordance with the restrictions of the simple case, these groups can be assured that every embryo is treated with the greatest respect and is put into the environment in which it has the best possible chance of surviving and growing into a baby.

Some IVF clinics scrupulously observe this restriction, never fertilizing more embryos than their patients will accept for transfer. The Jones's clinic in Norfolk, Virginia, is one that operates in this manner. Carl Wood's unit, on the other hand, fertilizes all the eggs they obtain; surplus embryos are normally frozen, though some eggs have been used in an egg donation programme. Should all IVF centres keep up with the Jones's, so far as respect for the embryos is concerned?

Neat as this way around a contentious ethical issue might be, we do not think it possible to avoid coming down on one side or the other in the dispute. For one thing, right-to-life groups are not always pacified by the assurance that all embryos created will be transferred to the womb. They point to the high rate of loss of the embryos, even when this is done. As we saw in Chapter 1, the survival rate per embryo transferred is still no higher than 18 per cent. Four out of five embryos created by the IVF programme are thus destined to die, even when they are all transferred to the womb. Admittedly, many eggs fertilized by natural sexual intercourse meet the same fate, failing to implant and dying in the first day or two after fertilization takes place. Nevertheless the rate of embryo loss in IVF is probably higher than in natural reproduction. Margaret Tighe, of Right to Life Australia, told us that she regards the natural loss of embryos as something that cannot be avoided; on the other hand the embryos lost during IVF are deliberately created in the knowledge that they will be exposed to high risks. Thus while she thought that putting all embryos into the womb was a definite improvement over the method used by Carl Wood, the improvement was not enough to make her fully accepting of IVF.

Even if right-to-life groups would accept IVF when all embryos are transferred to the womb, it would still be necessary to tackle the issue of the moral status of the embryo. There are advantages in creating more embryos than can be put into the womb. We saw in Chapter 1 that the chances of obtaining a pregnancy are much greater if three embryos are transferred than if only one or two are transferred. Although fertilization occurs on 90 per cent of the occasions on which a ripe egg and sperm are put together, and although in excess of 90 per cent of these fertilized eggs develop normally to the point at which they are ready for transfer to the womb, to be sure of having the right number of normal embryos for transfer on every occasion, it is necessary to attempt to fertilize more eggs than the number of embryos intended for transfer. On most occasions these attempts will all succeed, leaving more embryos than are wanted; the excess number fertilized is a safety margin for those occasions on which, for whatever reason, some eggs fail to be fertilized, or some embryos do not develop normally to the stage at which they are ready for transfer.

Another advantage of fertilizing more eggs than are needed is that it then becomes possible to select those embryos that appear to be growing best (the more rapidly cleaving embryos appear to have a higher rate of implantation). Nor should we forget the prospect of using the surplus embryos for research. Such research might be aimed at improving the pregnancy rates for IVF, at understanding the cause of some birth defects, or at providing materials for transplantation into injured or dying adults.

We shall say more about some of these prospects in Chapter 6. At this stage, two things are clear: first, that *if* an embryo has the same right to life as any human being, these uses of embryos are gravely wrong and ought to be strictly prohibited; second, that if we forego doing all these things because of a reluctance to confront the issue of the moral status of the embryo, we *might* be needlessly making it more difficult for IVF patients to have children, and needlessly giving up opportunities for research of great value not just for IVF but for medicine as a whole.

So the status of the embryo does matter. We cannot shelve the question, because to go ahead with work that leads to the destruction of embryos will be wrong if the embryo does have a moral status like more mature humans, and not to go ahead with such work will be a needless sacrifice if the embryo does not have this kind of status. The fundamental ethical question has to be resolved.

Many people find such questions bewildering. Seeing no way of answering them, they throw up their hands and say, 'It's all up to the individual's subjective judgement.' Our aim is to show that there is a rational answer to these questions, which should carry conviction with everyone who accepts one very widely held premise: that it is not wrong to destroy either the egg or the sperm before they have united.

On the basis of this premise we shall argue that there is no moral obligation to preserve the life of the embryo. Our argument applies specifically to the very early kind of embryo produced by the IVF programme. In other words, we are talking about an embryo that has developed for only some hours or at the most a day or two. It will only have divided a few times, into two, four, eight, or sixteen cells. At this stage, of course, the embryo has no brain, or even a nervous system. (Even the brain of a tadpole has more than 5,000 cells.) The embryo could not possibly feel anything or be conscious in any way. Therefore what we shall argue about this kind of embryo has no *necessary* application to an embryo at a later stage of development—for example, at a stage of development at which it does have a brain, and could feel pain.

Our argument begins from the premise that it is not wrong to destroy either the egg or the sperm—the gametes, as they are collectively known—before they have united. We do not know of anyone who seriously asserts that the moral status of the egg and sperm before fertilization is such that it is wrong to destroy them. For instance, if a man is asked to produce a specimen of semen so that it can be tested to see if he is fertile, no one objects to the semen being tipped out once the test is complete. And, after all, in our normal lives eggs and sperm are constantly being wasted. Every normal female between puberty and menopause wastes an egg each month that she does not become pregnant; and after puberty every normal male wastes millions of sperm in sexual intercourse in which contraceptives are used, or in which the woman is not fertile; and the same applies when he masturbates or has a nocturnal emission. Does anyone regard all this as a terrible tragedy? Not to our knowledge; and so we do not think the premise of our argument is likely to be challenged.

We shall consider some imaginary stories. They do not describe any actual occurrences or even probable ones. We are using them to illustrate a moral point.

First story

Doctors working on an IVF programme have obtained a fertile egg from a patient and some semen from the patient's husband. They are just about to drop the semen into the glass dish containing the egg, when the doctor in charge of the patient calls to say that he has discovered that she has a medical condition which makes pregnancy impossible. The egg could be fertilized and returned to the womb, but implantation would not occur. The embryo would die and be expelled during the woman's next monthly cycle. There is therefore no point in proceeding to fertilize the egg. So the egg and semen are tipped, separately, down the sink.

In accordance with our premise, as far as the moral status of the egg or the sperm before they have united is concerned, nothing wrong has been done.

Second story

Everything happens exactly as in the first story, except that the doctor in charge of the patient calls with the bad news *after* the egg and sperm have been placed in the glass dish and fertilization has already taken place. The couple are asked if they are prepared to consent to the newly created embryo being frozen to be implanted into someone else, but they are adamant that they do not want their genetic material to become someone else's child. Nor is there any prospect of the woman's condition ever changing, so there is no point in freezing the embryo in the hope of reimplanting it in her at a later date. The couple ask that the embryo be disposed of as soon as possible.

If the embryo has a special moral status that makes it wrong to destroy it, it would be wrong to comply with the couple's request. What, then, *should* be done with the embryo?

How plausible is the belief that it was not wrong to dispose of the egg and sperm separately but would be wrong to dispose of them after they have united? For those who believe that there is a real distinction between the two stories, here is a third story, not to be taken too seriously, but intended to bring out the peculiarity of that belief.

Third story

This story begins just as the first one does. The doctor's call comes before the egg and sperm have been united, and so they are tipped, separately, down the sink. But as luck would have it, the sink is blocked by a surgical dressing. As a result, the egg has not actually gone down the drain-pipe before the semen is thrown on top of it. A nurse is about to clear the blockage and flush them both away when a thought occurs to her: perhaps the egg has been fertilized by the semen that was thrown on top of it! If that has happened, or if there is even a significant chance of that having happened, those who believe that the embryo has a special moral status which makes it wrong to destroy it must now believe that it would be wrong to clear the blockage. Instead the egg must now be rescued from the sink, checked to see if fertilization has occurred, and if it has, efforts should presumably be made to keep it alive.

On what grounds could one try to defend the view that the coming together of the egg and sperm makes such a crucial difference to the way in which they ought to be treated? We shall consider three possible grounds which have been put forward.

(i) The claim that human life exists from conception

This claim is often used as an argument against abortion. We are not here considering the issue of abortion but rather the moral status of the embryo. Nevertheless, the claim is relevant to our topic because it is often assumed that once it is acknowledged that a human life exists from the moment of conception, it must be accepted that the embryo has the same basic right to life as normal human beings after birth.

To assess the claim that a human life exists from conception it is necessary to distinguish two possible senses of the term 'human being'. One sense is strictly biological: a human being is a member of the species *homo sapiens*. The other is more restricted: a human being is a being possessing, at least at a minimal level, the capacities distinctive of our species, which include consciousness, the ability to be aware of one's surroundings, the ability to relate to others, perhaps even rationality and self-consciousness.

When opponents of abortion say that the embryo is a living human being from conception onwards, all they can possibly mean is that the embryo is a living member of the species *homo sapiens*. This is all that can be established as a scientific fact. But is this also the sense in which every 'human being' has a right to life? We think not. To claim that every human being has a right to life solely because it is biologically a member of the species *homo sapiens* is to make species membership the basis of rights. This is as indefensible as making race membership the basis of rights. It is the form of prejudice one of us has elsewhere referred to as 'speciesism', a prejudice in favour of members of one's own species. The logic of this prejudice runs parallel to the logic of the racist who is prejudiced in favour of members of his race simply because they are members of his race. If we are to attribute rights on morally defensible grounds, we must base them on some morally relevant characteristic of the beings to whom we attribute rights. Examples of such morally relevant characteristics would be consciousness, autonomy, rationality, and so on, but not race or species.

Hence, although it may be possible to claim with strict literal accuracy that a human life exists from conception, it is not possible to claim that a human life exists from conception in the sense of a being which possesses, even at the most minimal level, the capacities distinctive of most human beings. Yet it is on the possession of these capacities that the attribution of a right to life, or of any other special moral status, must be based.

(ii) The claim from the potential of the embryo

It may be admitted that the embryo consisting of no more than sixteen cells cannot be said to be entitled to any special moral status because of the characteristics it actually possesses. It is, once again, far inferior to a tadpole in respect of all characteristics that could be regarded as morally relevant. But what of its potential? Unlike a tadpole, it has the potential to develop into a normal human being, with a high degree of rationality, self-consciousness, autonomy, and so on. Can this potential justify the belief that the embryo is entitled to a special moral status?

We believe that it cannot, for the following reason. Everything that can be said about the potential of the embryo can also be said about the potential of the egg and sperm when separate but considered jointly. If we have the egg and we have the sperm then what we have also has the potential to develop into a normal human being, with a high degree of rationality, self-consciousness, autonomy, and so on. On the basis of our premise that the egg and sperm separately have no special moral status, it seems impossible to use the potential of the embryo as a ground for giving it special moral status.

It is, of course, true that something may go wrong. The egg may be surrounded by semen, and yet not be fertilized. But it is also true that something may go wrong with the development of the embryo. It may fail to implant. It may implant but spontaneously abort. And so on. There is a possibility of something going wrong at every stage, from the production of egg and sperm right through to the time at which there is a rational and self-conscious being. That there is one more stage that the egg and sperm must go through, compared to the embryo, can scarcely make a decisive difference.

(iii) The uniqueness of the embryo

Some will concede that there is a sense in which the embryo, on the one hand, and the egg and sperm jointly, on the other hand, have the same potential, namely the potential to develop into a mature human being. Yet, they will want to say, there is a difference between these two forms of potential. As long as the egg and sperm are separate, the genetic nature of the individual human being that may come to exist is still to be determined. We have no way of telling which of the hundreds of thousands of sperm in a drop of semen will fertilize the egg. The unique genetic construction of the embryo, on the other hand, has been determined for all time. Can this difference provide a reason for giving the embryo higher status than the egg and sperm? Surely not, for the difference still does not show that the embryo has a different potential from the egg and sperm. Taken together the egg-and-sperm has the potential to develop into a mature human being. There are no genetically indeterminate human beings, and every genetically determinate human being is unique, with the exception of identical twins, triplets, and so on. Thus, the uniqueness of the embryo is nothing *additional* to its potential for becoming human. Why should our inability to tell which sperm will fertilize the egg make such a difference? If we were better able to predict which sperm would fertilize the egg, would we then say that the egg and sperm were now entitled to the same moral status as the embryo?

If it is uniqueness as such that we are talking about, and not the potential to develop into a mature human being, we should also remember that it is not only human beings who are genetically unique. Each individual chimpanzee is genetically unique too; so is each individual pig, and each individual rat, and each individual sparrow. Does that entitle them to special moral status? (Is it less evil to kill one of a pair of identical twins that it is to kill one of a pair of fraternal twins?)

Finally, if uniqueness is thought to be a basis for special moral status, what will happen when advances in the technique of cloning make it possible for each human cell to become an embryo? An embryo that is developed from the nucleus of a human cell in this manner would not be unique. Any other embryo developed in the same manner from a cell taken from the same person would be genetically identical to it. Would this mean that a cloned embryo would not have the moral status of a normal embryo? This seems an absurd conclusion; certainly it is one that cuts against all the other arguments we have been considering, for a cloned embryo is as much a living human being, and as much a potentially rational and self-conscious being, as a normal embryo.

Enter the soul

Behind these unsuccessful attempts to defend the special moral significance of conception in non-religious terms, there is often a more metaphysical belief: the belief that the soul enters the body at the point of conception.

Let us first of all spell out exactly what is being claimed by those who hold this view. They hold that for each human individual there is one and only one unique and indivisible spiritual substance or soul. It is not located in space, and since it is not a physical thing it can exist after the death of the physical body to which it is attached. Everyone has a soul, whether they know about it or not. It is what makes humans more significant than animals and is the immortal spark within each of us.

There are many standard objections to the philosophical claim that there are such things as souls. We will put these aside, however, since we don't need them for our very much more limited purpose of showing that, whether there are such things as souls or not, they certainly do not arrive at the point of conception. For consider again the occurrence of twinning. Nobody knows, when an egg is fertilized, whether it is subsequently going to divide and become identical twins or even triplets. It is also possible to divide the two-cell embryo surgically, thus creating deliberately a phenomenon which nature occasionally produces.

Obviously this generates problems for the doctrine that the soul arrives at conception. Souls can't split in two at the point that the embryo splits (or is divided) into identical twins. In the first place souls are not material objects and therefore cannot be split in two by a cellular division (or a cutting operation). In the second place we are told that souls are indivisible, and therefore cannot divide in two anyway. Perhaps it will be suggested that the soul does not divide, but stays with one of the two new cells, while a further soul is called into being for the benefit of the twin. But this would be a rather wild suggestion. Apart from the difficulty of determining which of the two identical cells was the 'new' one, and the consequent problem of there being a plausible candidate for retaining the 'old' soul, the suggestion involves the idea of a bizarre occurrence. We are familiar with the idea of the soul leaving the body, but if the soul arrived at conception, and the embryo subsequently split in two, one of the twins would have been involved in a process of the body leaving the soul. This would be no mean feat for a spatial object—to leave something that was not even physically present in space. Furthermore, by the definition of those who believe that the soul is attached to the body until death, the 'body' would die and return to life again when the new soul arrived. If this sounds like nonsense, it is; but it is nonsense that follows logically from the suggestion that the soul enters the body at the point of conception. When nonsense follows logically from any proposition whatever, the original proposition must itself be nonsense. If there are such things as souls, they do not arrive at the point of conception.

Do the same problems arise if it is suggested that the soul enters the body at a later point in development? No, they do not. Then when might the soul arrive? As soon as the possible cell divisions are safely out of the way and the metaphysical difficulties have disappeared? This would be arbitrary and perverse. The original belief that the soul enters the body at the point of conception was prompted by the fact that conception is a significant event in the determination of the future development of the genetic material. The division from two to four cells, or from four to eight, or from sixty-four to one hundred and twenty-eight, is not significant in anything like the same way. If there were such things as souls, the next plausible candidate for the point of arrival of the soul would be the point at which the embryo develops a rudimentary brain and becomes capable of sensation and feeling, as distinct from purely reflex movement.

The cut-off line

Since none of the grounds we have examined suffices to support a sharp distinction between the moral status of the embryo and that of the egg and sperm, we are left with just three possibilities: we must find another plausible reason for making this distinction; or we must abandon our initial premise, which was that the egg and sperm are not entitled to a special moral status which would make it wrong to destroy them; or we must hold that the embryo in its very earliest stage of life is also not entitled to a special moral status which would make it wrong to destroy it. We can find no other plausible reason for making the distinction. Our premise still seems well grounded. So we conclude that the newly created embryo is not entitled to a special moral status which makes it wrong to destroy it.

Our conclusion is contrary to the views of some pressure groups and of some theologians. On the other hand it is not at odds with the views of our community as a whole. There is little or no opposition to the use of intra-uterine devices (IUDs) as a means of preventing pregnancy. There is evidence that these devices often work not strictly as contraceptives; that is, not by preventing conception but by ensuring that any egg that is fertilized will fail to implant in the womb. The fertilized egg, or embryo, is then expelled from the womb and dies. If the embryo, from its earliest stages, were entitled to a special moral status which makes it wrong to kill it, the use of IUDs would be a serious violation of that special moral status.

We are not claiming that two wrongs make a right. We have argued that the embryo in its earliest stages does not have a special moral status that makes it wrong to kill it. Hence we do not think that it is wrong to use an IUD, or to discard any excess embryos produced by IVF techniques. We have mentioned IUDs only to make the point that anyone who objects to the disposal of excess embryos produced in the course of attempts at IVF should also, to be consistent, object just as strongly to the use of an IUD. Anyone who calls for a ban on the use of IVF because it may lead to the discarding of human embryos will be on very weak ground unless he or she also calls for a ban on the use of IUDs.

We put this point to Margaret Tighe, of Right to Life Australia. She agreed that IUDs result in the destruction of early embryos, and looked forward to the day when IUDs would not be used because they are incompatible with respect for human life. Mrs Tighe said that her campaign against abortion and IVF, based as it is on the principle of respect for life from the moment of conception, would, if successful, eventually lead to the introduction of laws which would also have the effect of prohibiting the use of the IUD. She said that abortion, which clearly kills a living being, and IVF, which with government funding was known to be deliberately creating human beings and just as deliberately destroying them, were at the present time a more urgent focus for her organization's campaign than the unknowable creation and loss of embryos through the use of the IUD.

The problem with this way of distinguishing the two situations is that while a fertile woman using an IUD and having normal sexual relations will not know precisely *when* her IUD destroys an embryo, she can know that over a long period of use, say a year, her IUD will almost certainly have destroyed at least one embryo, and probably more. Is that knowledge not sufficient to make the deliberate use of an IUD as culpable as the deliberate creation of embryos, some of which will not survive? Moreover if one were really concerned about the embryos themselves, rather than about the moral guilt of the agents involved, surely one would give priority to stopping the practice that causes the greater number of embryos to be destroyed—and the use of IUDs must be responsible for the deaths of several thousand times as many embryos as are lost through IVF.

The view we have argued for justifies the common-sense reaction which we believe most readers will have had to the three stories we told earlier. If you felt that it would be absurd to hold that the medical staff are under a moral obligation to try to rescue the egg that may have been accidentally fertilized in the blocked sink, you were right. Similarly, whether the doctor's call came a minute before the egg and sperm were to be united, or a minute afterwards, makes no crucial difference. In none of these cases has a being come into existence which is capable of feeling or experiencing anything at all. In none of these cases is there a being that has a right to life.

We have been able to resolve the issue of the moral status of the embryo. As far as rational moral argument is concerned, we can now conclude that there are no good reasons for avoiding procedures that lead to the creation of more embryos than can be transferred to the womb. The surplus embryos could be thrown out—if that was the wish of the medical team and the couple from whom the egg and sperm came—without infringing any rights, for the very early embryo is not yet a bearer of rights. Similarly, no rights of these very early embryos are violated when they are dissected or otherwise experimented upon for research purposes.

This discussion, and particularly the use of embryos for research, will naturally give rise to the question of when, in the course of normal development, the embryo does become a being that has rights. This question has always been asked of those who favour liberal abortion laws. Why should birth make a crucial difference? What qualities does a new-born baby possess that are not shared by the foetus after eight months of growth? The question is difficult to answer, especially if the comparison is between a late foetus and a very premature new-born.

We shall not try to provide a full answer to this question here, for to do so would take us too far from the issue of IVF. All we need to do is propose a safe minimal level, after which the embryo or foetus might plausibly be said to have some moral status which would make it wrong to carry out certain kinds of research.

We have said that while membership of a certain species is not a morally relevant characteristic, consciousness, autonomy, rationality, and so on, are. The most minimal of these is consciousness. As soon as a being becomes capable of feeling pleasure or pain, or of having experiences and preferring some kinds of experience to others, that being has sufficient moral status to make it wrong to do certain things to it, for example, to inflict pain upon it unnecessarily. Research on the embryo therefore ought to stop—or at least should only be permissible under extremely strict controls—as soon as the embryo reaches the stage at which it may be conscious.

But when does the embryo become conscious? Neither in embryos nor in adults do we observe consciousness directly—we infer it from behaviour, or from the degree of development of the nervous system. Scientists can examine the development of the embryo, but what kinds of behaviour and what degree of development of the nervous system indicates consciousness? We do not know. We can only look at the evidence, and speculate.

Here is some relevant evidence. Six weeks after conception, the embryo looks a bit like a curled-up tadpole, with a distinguishable head and tail. At this stage the central nervous system is beginning to form in a rudimentary manner, but it does not show the electrical activity characteristic of brain function in more developed beings. Nerve cells proper, and the chemical messengers that pass between them, do not form until eight weeks have passed. The 'higher' parts of the brain do not show any electrical activity, nor the nerve cell connections, until twelve weeks after conception. Meanwhile, between seven and eight weeks, the first response to stimuli, such as being touched around the mouth, has been observed; but it is not clear that this is anything more than a reflex. One expert in this area has concluded, after summarizing the available data, that the responses observed in foetuses less than eighteen weeks old are reflex activities that do not involve the parts of the brain associated with consciousness. A study of premature infants suggests that until about thirty-two weeks after

conception—or eight weeks before the time of normal birth—
sleep and wakefulness are difficult to distinguish, and the
premature infant is in a state of constant drowsiness.

Much more evidence could be brought forward, but it would
not settle the issue. We therefore make the following proposal.
The internationally recognized criterion for the permissibility of
using the vital parts of another human body is brain death. Total
brain death, the complete absence of all brain functions, indicates
that the heart, kidneys, the pancreas, and other organs may be
removed for transplant purposes. If the medical profession (and
indeed the Churches) recognize a body's lack of a functional
brain as sufficient grounds for declaring that there is no living
person existing in that body, and the body may therefore be used
as a means to worthwhile ends, then why not use the same
criterion at the other end of existence? We suggest that the
embryo be regarded as a thing, rather than a person, until the
point at which there is some brain function.

Brain function could not occur before the end of the sixth week
after conception; it may eventually be shown that it does not
occur until quite some time thereafter. We are happy to leave the
precise determination of the onset of brain function to the
scientists. As long as we proceed cautiously, choosing to err on
the side of safety, our criterion guarantees that nothing would be
done which infringed any rights the developing embryo might
plausibly be thought to have. No embryo would suffer by being
kept alive too long, nor by being experimented upon in a manner
that would cause it pain. Yet we could go ahead with IVF
procedures which involved the destruction of embryos a day or
two after conception; and research on the embryo would also be
possible, provided it was not carried beyond the point at which
the developing embryonic brain might begin to function.

Freezing embryos

When a Melbourne newspaper discovered that Carl Wood's IVF
team had frozen twelve surplus embryos, it broke the story with a
banner headline across the front page: 'Frozen Human Embryos'.
The tone of the story underneath was one of muted horror.

The freezing of embryos developed as a means of keeping the
surplus embryos which, as we have seen, are inevitably generated

by the use of fertility drugs. The freezing is done in liquid nitrogen, at a temperature of −196 degrees Celsius. At this temperature the embryos can remain frozen, without deteriorating, virtually indefinitely—six hundred years, according to one estimate.

Edwards and Steptoe tried to freeze 'spare' embryos as early as 1977, before Louise Brown had been born, but they could not get them to grow after thawing, and the experiment was discontinued. Alan Trounson, the scientific director of Carl Wood's team, had worked on the freezing of cattle embryos at Cambridge University before joining the IVF unit in Melbourne. At Cambridge he had found that passing the embryos through a special solution protected the cells against being ruptured by ice crystals. Therefore in 1980 Trounson, together with Wood and Leeton, approached the Queen Victoria Hospital Ethics Committee with the proposal that surplus embryos from the IVF programme should be frozen for later use. The committee agreed that freezing was preferable to disposing of the excess embryos or using them for research. Freezing began immediately, and the team was soon able to thaw embryos which continued to develop in culture after thawing. They began transferring these thawed embryos to the patients who had donated them.

Despite the initial success in freezing and thawing, the first embryos transferred did not implant. It was not until May 1983, after more than a dozen unsuccessful attempts, that Wood's team was able to announce the world's first pregnancy from an embryo that had been frozen. The pregnancy was to an unnamed Victorian woman, infertile because of blocked Fallopian tubes. She had had four eggs collected and fertilized as part of normal IVF treatment in 1982. Three embryos had been transferred 'fresh' and the fourth was frozen at the eight-cell stage. A pregnancy did result from the initial transfer, but it miscarried at eight weeks. The woman and her husband then asked for the fourth embryo, now 'on ice' for four months, to be thawed and transferred at the right moment of the woman's natural ovulatory cycle. On thawing, it was found that two of the eight cells of the embryo had been ruptured by the freezing process; nevertheless Trounson was sufficiently confident of the recuperative ability of such early embryos to go ahead. His studies on other species had convinced him that an embryo can have damage to several cells and still develop normally, because at this stage other cells take over the role that would have been played by the damaged ones. Unfortunately this pregnancy miscarried too, after twenty-four weeks. Subsequent tests showed, however, that the foetus was normal and that the miscarriage was not related to the freeze–thaw technique.

The Queen Victoria Hospital Ethics Committee accepted the freezing of embryos because this is less drastic than throwing them out. The argument of our previous section suggests that if the parties involved wished to do so, there would be no ethical barrier to destroying the embryos; nevertheless freezing may well be the wiser course, from a political point of view.

The development of embryo freezing can also be defended as a means of reducing the number of egg collections that IVF patients have to undergo. The egg collection is the most invasive part of the IVF procedure, for cuts have to be made, under anaesthesia, in the abdominal wall for the insertion of the laparoscope, forceps, and the needle through which the egg is siphoned out. If eight eggs are collected in one operation and all are fertilized, no more than two or three would be transferred back at any one time. The transfer, though a relatively simple step, not requiring any surgery, has the lowest success rate of any part of the IVF procedure. Without freezing, if the transfer fails, the patient will need to undergo another egg collection; but if embryos can be frozen and then thawed and successfully implanted in the womb, embryos left over after the first transfer can be used later in a second or third attempt. (Freezing the eggs and sperm separately would have the same effect, but to date it has proved impossible to freeze human eggs without destroying them.)

Even without the use of fertility drugs, IVF centres would find freezing useful on some occasions. It can happen that after the eggs are collected, the patient bleeds from the uterus, or becomes ill. Then the embryos cannot be transferred. Without freezing, they would have to be discarded or used for research. The patient would then need to have her eggs collected again at a later date. With freezing, the date of the transfer would simply be postponed. Long-term embryo freezing might also enable a woman to have her children relatively late in life—say when she was forty—without the increased risk of genetic defect that this normally involves.

Is there any ethical objection to freezing? Right-to-life groups, of course, have objected to the production of surplus embryos which has led to the 'freeze or discard' dilemma. They see freezing as reckless experimentation with human life. The Roman Catholic Archbishop of Melbourne has taken a similar hostile stance. The general public is less sure. The Morgan poll conducted in Australia in July 1982 asked the following questions:

With the test-tube method, it's possible for several eggs to be collected from a woman, and fertilized with her husband's sperm. Sometimes not all of those fertilized eggs are used. It's been suggested that fertilized eggs not used should be frozen for the couple to use for a later pregnancy. Do you approve or disapprove of that?

Of the Australian sample 44 per cent approved, and 33 per cent disapproved. The remainder said they needed to know more, or had no opinion. The same question was asked two months later in Britain, and here—possibly because freezing has not been attempted in Britain—the reaction was different. Only 38 per cent approved, with 45 per cent disapproving.

If we are right about the moral status of the embryo, the opposition of right-to-life groups and the Roman Catholic Church is ill-founded. That few embryos have survived freezing does not make freezing wrong. There is, however, one remaining source of anxiety which is not so easily overcome. This is the possibility that freezing may produce a higher rate of abnormalities. Clifford Grobstein has pointed out that while a 90 per cent success rate may be acceptable when we are dealing with frozen cattle or mice embryos, it would be a disaster in humans if the failures are not detectable until birth or even later. This worry is similar to that expressed about IVF as a whole. As we saw in the previous chapter, doubts about the safety of IVF in the simple case are receding as the number of normal children increases. Freezing, though, is a separate issue, with its own risks. Whether these risks are worth running depends on how great the risk might be, and the gains to be achieved if the procedure works.

We are not sufficiently expert in cryobiology—the science of freezing organic materials—to assess the risk of abnormalities resulting from the freezing of human embryos. Trounson believes that there is no risk—either the damage will be so severe that the embryo will not survive, or it will develop normally. At this early stage, Trounson believes, nature eliminates the mistakes. Edwards shares this view, which is supported by the results of freezing and thawing thousands of mouse, rat, cattle, and sheep embryos. With these animals, there has been no unusual rate of abnormalities.

Against this confidence in the safety of the procedure, one has to balance the fact that the gains to be made from freezing cannot compare with the gains from IVF as a whole. Unlike IVF itself, freezing is not the only way of enabling an infertile couple to have their much wanted child. It is, rather, a way of avoiding the need to repeat the minor, but safe, egg collection operation. Is this worth any risk, however slight, to the offspring?

Because of the difficulty in assessing whether freezing does pose even the slightest added risk of an abnormal child, we believe that the decision to use a frozen embryo should be made by the couple and the doctors, after discussion of the possibility that some unknown factor may increase the risk of abnormalities. Only the couple themselves can judge the importance to them of avoiding another operation for egg collection. Naturally, any resulting pregnancies should be carefully monitored and an abortion offered if a defect is revealed. Freezing should be used sparingly until there has been an opportunity to examine the first few children to develop from frozen embryos.

The remaining ethical issue is how long embryos should be kept frozen. Should long-term embryo freezing become a reality, a child might be born a century or more after the death of its genetic parents. The child would grow up among the great-great-grandchildren of its genetic brothers and sisters. Would this matter? Perhaps it sounds more bizarre than it would prove to be in real life. The Australian National Health and Medical Research Council has considered this issue, and said that there should be a maximum storage time of ten years, and in any case not longer than the 'time of conventional reproductive need or competence of the female donor'. Presumably this suggestion is intended to avoid the problem of what to do with frozen embryos whose genetic parents have passed the period at which they can reproduce, or have died. The council of the British Medical Association, in its report on IVF, set a much tighter time limit: 'Storage should not exceed 12 months, and the couple's wishes in relation to ultimate disposal should, as far as possible, be respected.'

The view of the British Medical Association invites an obvious retort: what if, after twelve months, the wishes of the couple are that the embryo remain frozen? We side with the right of the couple to make the decisions, rather than with arbitrary time limits. As we saw earlier, these embryos do not have a moral status superior to that of the egg and the sperm. The essential questions are not to do with the right to life of the frozen embryos, but rather with ensuring that the wishes of the couples are clearly stated at the time the embryo is frozen. These wishes should cover all foreseeable eventualities. The other important issue is the welfare of the future child, if the embryo is going to be allowed to develop into a child.

There seems no reason to believe that couples are unable to express their intentions for the fate of their embryos in various possible situations. In our questionnaire we asked couples on the IVF programme who should make decisions for the use of a frozen embryo if an IVF couple were to separate or divorce. By 83 per cent to 11 per cent, with 6 per cent undecided, they agreed with the statement: 'Both parties must consent to any use of embryos.' When asked who should make decisions about the use of any frozen embryos if both members of the couple should die, 67 per cent agreed with leaving the decision to the IVF team, with 21 per cent against.

Admittedly, there are legal problems here which need to be clarified. Is the embryo the property of the couple concerned? We asked the couples whether they considered it was: 90 per cent said they did. They may not, however, have considered the legal problems of a property approach. In law, if the joint owners of property disagree as to what is to be done with it, the courts have several accepted remedies: they can order it to be equally divided; they can order it to be sold, and the proceeds of the sale equally divided; or they can allow one of the two joint owners to retain the property, and pay half its value to the other. None of these remedies seems altogether appropriate here. Surprisingly—

especially for those who think of embryos as tiny babies—King Solomon's remedy of equal division might well be the best of this lot. At this early stage, each surgically separated half would be able to develop normally—thus each partner would have one of a pair of identical twin embryos. (For further details, see Chapter 6.)

That would be one possible solution; the alternative is to abandon the idea that the embryo is property, and instead consider it as a potential future child. Then the dispute could be seen as one over custody—a familiar enough problem for the courts, if one that rarely has an ideal solution. Mr Justice Asche, of the Family Court of Australia, has stated that the custody model might be the best way of reaching a solution. It need not depend, he maintains, on the court first ruling on whether or not the embryo is a legal person. The law would simply be applying a general principle to the circumstances before it.

We shall not attempt to predict the evolution of the law in this new area. New solutions will have to be found to unusual problems. For most couples, however, the problems will not arise. If a couple have been well counselled and have signed statements covering the most likely eventualities, few of these disputes should need to go to court to be resolved.

PART II
Looking Ahead

4 SURROGATE MOTHERHOOD

The past

A surrogate is a person or thing that acts for, or takes the place of, another. A surrogate mother, as the term is now used, is a woman who acts for another woman by having a child for her. The exact sense in which the surrogate has a child 'for' another woman can vary, as we shall see; but there is nothing new about the basic idea of surrogate motherhood. It is even in the Bible. The sixteenth chapter of Genesis tells the following story about Abraham and his wife Sarah (who have, at this stage, not yet been given the new names they receive from God after he makes his covenant with Abraham, and hence are referred to by their original names of Abram and Sarai):

Abram's wife Sarai had borne him no children. Now she had an Egyptian slave-girl whose name was Hagar, and she said to Abram, 'You see that the Lord has not allowed me to bear a child. Take my slave-girl; perhaps I shall found a family through her.' Abram agreed to what his wife said, so Sarai, Abram's wife, brought her slave-girl, Hagar the Egyptian, and gave her to her husband Abram as a wife . . . He lay with Hagar and she conceived . . .

This particular episode of surrogate motherhood worked out all right in the end, but it was not without its ups and downs. When Hagar knew that she had conceived, she began to despise her barren mistress. Sarai, knowing this, dealt so severely with Hagar that the pregnant maid fled into the wilderness. There God came to her and persuaded her to return, telling her that her child would be a son, Ishmael. Ishmael was duly born, but he had his own troubles. When God made his covenant with Abram, he promised to bless Sarai with a son. Though Sarah, as she was now called, was well past menopause, the Lord fulfilled his pledge, and she gave birth to Isaac. Sarah then told Abraham to cast out Ishmael, because she did not want the son of her servant to be his heir along with her own son. Abraham grieved at the thought of sending away one of his sons, but God said that he should do as Sarah had asked; consoling him by saying that although Isaac would pass on Abraham's line of descent, Ishmael too would be the founder of a nation. Ishmael survived to be the father of twelve princes, and to die at a ripe old age.

Surrogate motherhood may not have been uncommon among the ancient Hebrews. A second instance is described in the thirtieth chapter of Genesis. When Rachel found that she bore Jacob no children, she told him to lie with her slave-girl, Bilhah, 'so that she may bear sons to be laid upon my knees, and through her I too may build up a family'. Jacob dutifully followed her instructions, and had two sons from Bilhah. Nor is this the end of the story. Rachel was not Jacob's only wife. He had been forced, by the custom of the land in which he was staying, to marry her older sister, Leah, as well. Leah bore Jacob four sons; and it was because Rachel envied her sister, whom she obviously saw as some kind of rival for her husband's affections, that Rachel wished Jacob to have children with her maid. But when Leah saw that Jacob had sons from Bilhah, and that she herself had 'left bearing', she took her own slave-girl, Zilpah, and gave her to Jacob, who conceived another two sons with her. And as if that wasn't enough for Jacob, Leah then began to bear again, and had two more sons and a daughter. Meanwhile God belatedly heard Rachel's prayer, and she bore Jacob two sons as well.

The present

Abram and Sarai, and Jacob and his wives, needed no modern technology for their ventures into surrogate motherhood. Of course, a child like Ishmael, for instance, was not Sarai's child in any biological sense, even though Sarai might have thought of him as 'hers' (until she gave birth to a child that really was hers). Sarai could regard the child as hers because Hagar was her slave and so Sarai could 'found a family through her'. The same would have been true of Rachel and Leah, and the children of their slaves.

Freedom of contract and the market-place have now replaced slavery in civilized nations; and this applies to surrogate motherhood as well. Here is how the twentieth-century American equivalents of Abram, Sarai, and Hagar solved their problem.

Stefan was forty-three and his wife, Nadia, was thirty-nine (the names are fictitious, but the people and events real). For eighteen years they had wanted children, but Nadia's Fallopian tubes were blocked. Four major operations achieved nothing except an ectopic pregnancy. After a further operation, her doctor told her that she would never become pregnant. She sought a second opinion. The second doctor told her to give up. Soon after, the couple heard about the 'test-tube' baby born in Britain. They wrote to Edwards and Steptoe, but were told that women over thirty-six were not taken onto the programme. When the first American IVF clinic started up in Virginia they inquired again, only to be told once more that they were too old. Then in 1980 they heard about Noel Keane, a Michigan lawyer who arranges contracts between infertile couples and women who are prepared to act as surrogate mothers.

They went to see Keane, who explained that Michigan state laws prohibited the payment of a fee to a surrogate mother—and without offering a fee it could take a long time to find a woman who would act as a surrogate. In Kentucky, however, a fee could legally be paid. Moreover a Kentucky doctor, Richard Levin, had recently set up Surrogate Parenting Associates, Inc., to handle just this sort of case. Keane offered to refer them to Levin, but explained that in addition to establishing legal residence in Kentucky, they would have to find at least $22,000; $10,000 for the surrogate mother's fee, $5,000 for her medical expenses, $5,000 for legal fees to draw up the contract and arrange the eventual adoption, and $2,000 for 'miscellaneous expenses'.

The cost did not deter Stefan and Nadia, who saw this as their last hope of a child. They told Keane to go ahead. He arranged for an advertisement seeking a surrogate mother to be placed in a major Kentucky newspaper. Several potential surrogate mothers responded. They were interviewed by staff at Surrogate Parenting Associates, who then asked Stefan and Nadia to make their choice on the basis of information about the women's physical characteristics, health, religion, ethnic background, education, and other insights gained from the interviews. When the surrogate had been selected, she signed a contract with Surrogate Parenting, agreeing to turn the child over to the biological father at birth, and to allow it to be adopted by his wife. Another clause in the contract required her not to smoke or to take alcohol or other drugs during the pregnancy. In turn Stefan and Nadia had to put $10,000 in deposit for the surrogate mother to receive when she handed over the child. Then the surrogate mother was artificially inseminated with Stefan's sperm. To the delight of Stefan and Nadia she soon became pregnant. Their child was on its way at last.

The future

The child Stefan and Nadia will bring up as their own is not, genetically, *their* child. Like Hagar, the surrogate mother will have contributed half the genetic make-up of the child; and like Sarai, Nadia will have no genetic relationship to the child. Thus while the surrogate mother does, in uniting her egg with Stefan's sperm and bringing Stefan's child into the world, act as a surrogate for Nadia, she is no *mere* surrogate mother: she is, indisputably and unalterably, the true genetic mother of the child Nadia has adopted. For infertile women from the time of Sarai until the present time, there has been no way of overcoming this drawback to the use of another woman to bear the wanted child.

Now the technology of *in vitro* fertilization promises to change this situation entirely. An infertile woman who is producing eggs could have one or more of her eggs removed, fertilized with her husband's sperm, and then transferred into the womb of the surrogate mother. If the transfer were successful the surrogate mother would experience a normal pregnancy, but the baby that would emerge from her womb at the end of the pregnancy would not be her baby in the genetic sense. After birth the surrogate would hand the baby over to its genetic parents, who had supplied the egg and sperm, and the genetic parents would bring the child up as their own—which it would indeed be.

This is a true surrogate pregnancy. The surrogate provides nothing but the use of her body as a place in which the embryo can grow and be nourished. It is to this procedure—not to the method used by Surrogate Parenting Associates—that the journalists' nickname 'rent-a-womb', might without too great a distortion, be applied. We shall call this form of surrogacy, which makes use of *in vitro* fertilization, 'full surrogacy'; we shall thus distinguish it from 'partial surrogacy' which uses either natural intercourse or artificial insemination, and in which as a result the surrogate is also the genetic mother of the child she gives up.

At the time of writing no cases of full surrogacy have been reported, and leading IVF teams have said that they would not attempt to transfer an embryo to a surrogate. In 1981 Carl Wood's team announced that several Victorian women had volunteered to act as surrogate mothers for couples unable to have children. The question was put to the ethics committee of the Queen Victoria Medical Centre, where the team is based. After some deliberation, the committee instructed the IVF team not to attempt to make a surrogate pregnant. No reasons were given, beyond a statement by the general manager of the medical centre that the legal and ethical implications of surrogate motherhood were 'about as grey as you can get'.

The following year, the Australian National Health and Medical Research Council issued its guide-lines on IVF, and also put surrogate motherhood into the 'grey' category. 'Because of current inability to determine or define motherhood in this context,' it said, 'this situation is not yet capable of ethical resolution.' A year later, the British Medical Association's working party on IVF reported in similarly indecisive terms: 'The working group has yet to be satisfied that to undertake *in vitro* fertilization with the sperm and the ova of a couple and to transfer the embryo to the uterus of another woman who might carry the embryo to term on behalf of the couple will ever be acceptable.'

So for the moment, it seems that full surrogate motherhood is out, at least in Australia and Britain. Strictly from a technical point of view, however, there is no doubt that IVF has reached the point at which full surrogacy could be achieved. The procedure would require that the cycles of the two women be synchronized, but this could be done by administering hormones. Alternatively, the embryo could be frozen and then thawed when the surrogate was ready to have it implanted. As we saw in the previous chapter, Carl Wood's team succeeded in obtaining a pregnancy—albeit a short-lived one—from a donated egg and sperm. In this instance the intention of all the parties was that the woman receiving the embryo should keep the baby and bring it up as her own. She was not therefore acting as a surrogate. But presumably the prospects of the embryo implanting are not affected by whether the woman intends to keep the baby or to hand it over to its genetic parents. So this case of the successful implantation of a donor embryo makes it virtually certain that full surrogate motherhood could be achieved now if one of the leading IVF teams were to attempt it.

Reasons for surrogacy

Why would a couple seek a surrogate? Nadia could not have children because her tubes were blocked; IVF alone might have overcome that problem, and if Nadia had been accepted by an IVF clinic she would not have needed a surrogate. Now that IVF is becoming more widely available, Nadia's age would be less of an obstacle to IVF treatment. So couples like Stefan and Nadia are not, in the long run, going to be the people interested in finding a woman to act as a full surrogate.

The initial demand will come from women who are physically incapable of pregnancy, whether by normal means or by IVF. The most obvious candidates are women who have had diseased wombs which had to be removed. Such women may still have intact ovaries producing eggs in the normal manner, but their only hope of having one of these eggs grow into a child is for it to be surgically removed, fertilized in the laboratory, and then transferred into the womb of a woman prepared to act as a surrogate.

There are other medical conditions which make pregnancy dangerous rather than totally impossible: kidney disease, for instance, or drug-resistant high blood pressure. Here a woman would normally have to choose between giving up her desire for her own child, and becoming pregnant in the knowledge that for her, pregnancy may shorten her life. The use of a surrogate would be a way around this agonizing dilemma.

These reasons for seeking a surrogate mother are similar to the reasons why couples now seek IVF: it offers the only chance of a child that has a genetic relationship to the couple; and where adoption is not available, it offers the only chance the couple have of any sort of child. The use of surrogacy in these situations can therefore be regarded as a medical response to a defect in the woman's reproductive system or to a defect in her general health that makes pregnancy inadvisable.

Surrogacy might also be sought for quite different reasons. The time when many couples wish to begin a family coincides, for some women, with an important stage of their career. If pregnancy would interrupt a woman's career, perhaps leaving her permanently behind her male colleagues of the same age, a woman might want someone else to carry the embryo for her, so that she could continue her career and still have her baby. Other women might wish to avoid pregnancy because of the effect it has on their figures. For a model this could be a matter of continuing her career; for other women the motivation might be aesthetic, or perhaps a matter of attractiveness to men. Some women simply would rather do without the prospect of morning sickness and several months of feeling large and heavy, followed by the pain of childbirth.

Reasons for surrogacy thus range all the way from straightforward medical indications to what one might regard as 'mere convenience'. Nor is there any easy way of drawing a line between the two: rather there is a gradual continuum stretching from those women who physically cannot have a child without surrogacy; through those who can have a child in the normal manner but only at some risk to their lives; to those who may have more minor health grounds for avoiding pregnancy (perhaps it will aggravate their varicose veins); and to those who have serious professional considerations against becoming pregnant; and finally to those who have only those reasons against pregnancy that every woman could have, if she were inclined to give them sufficient weight.

In this situation, one approach would be to insist on a line being drawn somewhere, no matter how difficult the task. Just as, one might say, the State must somehow decide when surgery is medically indicated and therefore to be subsidized by public funds, and when surgery is purely cosmetic and therefore to be paid for privately if it is to be done at all; so the State must somehow decide which requests for surrogate motherhood are medically indicated and should therefore go ahead, and which cases are entirely optional and therefore should not go ahead. In borderline cases there may be some arbitrariness about such decisions, but once a few precedents have been established, the great majority of cases will fall clearly on one or other side of the line.

Advocates of a free market with minimal State interference would object to this approach. They would claim that the market, not the State, should be allowed to determine when surrogacy is to be available. Any other approach, they would say, infringes on the freedom of individuals to buy and sell as they choose. On this view, if someone seeking a surrogate can afford to pay enough to persuade another woman to act as a surrogate for her, she should be free to go ahead at her own expense, no matter how silly or trivial her reasons for wanting to avoid pregnancy may be.

We noted this type of argument in the previous chapter, when we raised the question whether sperm and egg donors should be paid. In that case it seemed likely that enough people would be willing to donate without payment, other than perhaps a modest compensation for any inconvenience involved in the donation. The question of a right to trade in eggs and sperm we therefore did not discuss in any detail, for we saw practical advantages in a non-commercial system. With surrogacy, however, the situation is different. Bearing a child is a major undertaking, at least when compared to donating sperm or an egg. The fees offered for this service can be expected to be correspondingly large. Stefan and Nadia were, as we saw, prepared to pay $22,000 for a partial surrogate; of this, $10,000 was for the surrogate herself. Hence there is some point to the claim that a State prohibition of a free market in surrogate services would be a serious restriction on the right of the potential surrogate to earn her living in the way she chooses, and an equally serious restriction on the right of the surrogate-seeking couple to offer a price sufficient to attract those willing to provide the service they seek. Whatever point this claim has, however, must be set against objections to surrogacy in general and to commercial surrogacy in particular.

Objections to surrogacy

Surrogate motherhood is one of the few applications of IVF of which the general public disapproves. That, at least, is the finding of the 1982 Morgan Gallup Poll in Australia and in

Britain. After people had answered questions about more straightforward uses of IVF, they were told the following:

The fertilized egg from one married couple could be put into *another* woman, who would then become pregnant. She would *give the baby back* to the couple after it was born.

More than 70 per cent of the sample in each country said they had heard about this procedure. They were then asked:

Do you think this sort of test-tube baby treatment for married couples to have a child by *another* woman should be *allowed*, or *not*?

In Australia, 32 per cent thought it should be allowed, but 44 per cent thought it should not be. In Britain only 20 per cent thought it should be allowed, with a solid majority of 55 per cent against allowing it. In both countries around a quarter of respondents either had no opinion, or said that they needed to know more, or that the answer depended on other factors.

The poll data does not tell us why so many people thought that full surrogate motherhood should not be allowed. The response is a contrast to the more approving reaction we noted in the previous chapter to the question about the donation of fertilized eggs—or 'pre-natal adoption'. One reason for this different response might be that people do not like the idea of a woman having to 'give back' a baby to whom she has given birth. We shall see in a moment that there is some reason for concern about this aspect of surrogate motherhood. But there is also a crucial difference in the way the two questions were put, which makes the answers not strictly comparable. When people were asked about the donation of fertilized eggs, they were told that the eggs were to be given to another married couple 'so that they can have a child'. The clear implication is that the married couple to whom the eggs are given could not have a child by any other method. In the question asked about surrogate motherhood there was no such implication. Respondents therefore may not have had the plight of the childless couple in mind when they answered. It was open to them to interpret the question as one about a married couple who could have children by the normal method but find it more convenient to use a surrogate. If some respondents did interpret the question in this way, the negative response is easily explained.

No doubt a significant number of people do oppose surrogate motherhood even for couples who cannot otherwise have children. Some may think of it as unnatural, and for that reason wrong. We shall not repeat here the arguments we used in Chapter 2 concerning what is natural and what is not. We will simply repeat our conclusion that the naturalness or unnaturalness of a new procedure is not the real issue: the crucial question is whether the procedure is likely to do more good than harm.

Here opponents of surrogacy will point to the horrendous legal tangles that could arise with full surrogacy. Some of these tangles have already arisen among the relatively small number of partial surrogacy arrangements made so far. Although partial surrogacy differs in some relevant respects from full surrogacy, the problems that have arisen with partial surrogacy are at present the best guide to the likely problems of full surrogacy.

Noel Keane, the American lawyer who helped Stefan and Nadia arrange their partial surrogacy contract, has written a book, *The Surrogate Mother*, describing his work in this new field. Keane credits himself with the path-breaking legal work that has made partial surrogacy a reality for many infertile couples. There is no doubt about his enthusiasm for surrogacy. 'Surrogate parenting', he tells us, 'is an idea whose time is coming . . . I think it will replace adoption.' The book itself, Keane says, 'is my legal brief on behalf of a controversial cause to make surrogate motherhood a common reality in the years ahead'.

Given Keane's advocacy of the cause, some sections of *The Surrogate Mother* are alarming. Perhaps most dramatic is the story of Bill and Bridget. In fairness to Keane, it has to be said that the case was one of his early ones. It began in 1977, before he quite knew what he was getting into; nevertheless it illustrates some possible pitfalls of surrogacy.

Bill and Bridget were an infertile couple. Keane put them in touch with Diane. Diane had seen a television talk show in which Keane appeared with another infertile couple and their pregnant partial surrogate. After the show, Diane had phoned offering to help a couple to have a child. She was a thirty-one-year-old divorcee, living in Tennessee with a two-year-old son: when interviewed she seemed a good mother and responsible parent. At that time Keane had not discovered that Kentucky State law allowed the payment of a fee to surrogate mothers, so Diane was told that nothing could be paid except expenses. She signed an agreement to that effect.

Diane soon became pregnant with Bill's child. Then things began to go wrong. She asked Bill and Bridget for money to travel to Boston to visit her mother. They sent her the money. She said she had been robbed of expense money they had sent her. They sent her another cheque. Then her car needed repairs, she had extra medical expenses . . . and so on. Often when she phoned asking for money, she sounded drunk or stoned on drugs. Sometimes she threatened to kill herself unless she got more money. Bill and Bridget did not dare call her bluff. Shortly before the baby was due, Diane demanded $3,000 to pay for a computer course she planned to take. Bill and Bridget paid. In all, they calculated that they sent Diane more than $12,000.

Finally, two weeks before the due date, Diane phoned to say that she was in jail on a drunk-driving charge, and needed bail money. Bill and Bridget flew to Tennessee to stay with Diane and try to prevent anything else going wrong before she had the baby. That is when that found that Diane's 'roommate', Vicky, was really her lover. In despair Bridget turned on her husband. 'Bill', she screamed, 'do you realize that the woman you got pregnant is not only an alcoholic and drug addict but also a lesbian!'

Amazingly, the story has a happy ending. Diane gave birth to a boy, below normal weight and suffering from drug withdrawal symptoms; but after five days in hospital Bill, Jr. was healthy enough to go home with his father and his new mother. Diane tried for some time to extract more money by threatening to hold up the adoption proceeding; but when this threat failed to have any effect, she moved interstate without leaving any forwarding address. At the time of writing Keane described the child as 'in legal limbo', but Bill and Bridget were so happy with 'their' child that they told Keane: 'He has made it all worthwhile.'

Two other bizarre Keane stories ended less happily. The first, related in *The Surrogate Mother*, concerns John and Lorelei, a married Connecticut couple unable to have children. The usual story, except that in this case the infertility was not unexpected:

Lorelei was a transsexual. Until the age of twenty-one, she had been male. For Keane, this was no obstacle. He took the couple on as his clients. They found Rita, a divorced Californian mother of three who said she was interested in being a surrogate mother 'for humanitarian reasons'. Rita became pregnant, and then asked for $7,500. Keane advised John and Lorelei that they would be breaking the law if they paid; in any case they could not afford to pay. They refused. Rita wrote back: 'I have decided to keep my baby, and the deal is off.'

The baby, a boy, was born in April 1981. Keane brought a custody suit on behalf of John. Blood tests showed with 99 per cent probability that he was the father. Before the case came to court, however, it became apparent that Lorelei's transsexualism would come out into the open and probably damage their already slim chances of success. In a vain atempt to avoid publicity, John and Lorelei decided to give up the legal battle for custody.

Our final Keane disaster is not taken from the pages of his book. It was, however, anticipated by a prescient quotation in the book, taken from an editorial in the *Detroit News*. Writing of the possible legal dilemmas of the new method of motherhood, the editorial asked:

What happens if the proxy mother gives birth to a defective child and the couple refuses to adopt it? Can the surrogate mother sue the father for damages arising from pregnancy? How can the husband be sure he is indeed the father of his 'investment', short of isolating the surrogate from other male contacts?

Keane did not answer these questions in *The Surrogate Mother*. Soon after the book appeared, however, he found himself unable to avoid them.

Late in 1981 Judy Stiver, a Michigan housewife, noticed an advertisement in a local paper. It was one placed regularly by Keane, and it sought women willing to become surrogate mothers for a fee. Judy and her husband, Ray, had a two-year-old daughter, and going through pregnancy again seemed a good way to earn some extra cash. 'We wanted the money to pay some bills and take a vacation', she explained later to a reporter.

Through Keane, Judy Stiver met Alexander and Nadia Malahoff, of New York. She agreed to be impregnated with

Alexander Malahoff's sperm and to abstain from sexual intercourse until the baby was conceived. In return, Malahoff agreed
to take the baby and pay Mrs Stiver $10,000. All went well until
the baby was born, when it was discovered that he suffered from
microcephaly, a condition in which the head is abnormally small,
and the child often turns out to be mentally retarded.

At first the child was not expected to live: when it became
apparent that he would, Malahoff claimed that the baby's blood
tests showed that he could not have been the father. Accordingly
he refused to accept the baby, and to pay Judy Stiver the agreed
fee. At first the Stivers also refused to take the baby, saying that
they had come to accept that the baby would be taken from Mrs
Stiver, and they did not want another child. When further court-
ordered blood tests confirmed that Alexander Malahoff was not
the father, however, the Stivers finally agreed to keep the baby.

Many people would consider these episodes provide sufficient
grounds for prohibiting surrogacy, whether partial or full. Once
we mess around with conventional arrangements for bearing and
rearing children, there is no end to the complications that can
arise. The result is distress for all concerned.

To those who argue that couples and would-be surrogates have
the right to make their own private contractual arrangements in
matters that concern no one else, the opponents of surrogacy
could reply that in surrogacy contracts someone else is always
affected: the child. Society has a right, they would claim, to
prohibit such arrangements in order to prevent children being
born in undesirable circumstances. They might add that the
childless couple are usually too desperate to take proper steps to
ensure that a woman offering to act as a surrogate really is a fit
and proper person for that purpose. The story of Bill and Bridget
suggests this; and Lorelei told Keane that when Rita offered to
act as a surrogate, 'we were so excited we would have taken
someone with purple skin from Mozambique'.

Discussion

We have seen that when A and B have a surrogate motherhood
contract with C, at least four things are liable to go wrong:

(1) C might have contracted to refrain from taking alcohol or drugs, but
    might do it anyway.

(2) C might, during pregnancy, attempt to extort payment, or additional payment beyond any agreed fee, from A and B. To do this she might threaten to have an abortion, or to keep the baby.

(3) C might decide, once the baby is born, that she wishes to keep it, in spite of her contract to give it to A and B.

(4) A and B might decide, once the baby is born, that they do not wish to accept it, perhaps because it is born with a handicap, perhaps because they do not believe it is their genetic child.

No doubt there are many other complications that could arise, but these instances are enough to indicate where surrogacy can lead.

No one denies that surrogacy can cause problems—least of all Keane, who has to be given credit for having openly displayed the troubles some of his clients found themselves in. Keane does not, of course, believe that the problems are a reason for prohibiting surrogacy. He would point to the cases like that of Stefan and Nadia, in which a surrogacy agreement went smoothly, leaving a couple ecstatic over the fulfilment of their otherwise impossible dream of having a child, and a surrogate mother happy with her fee, or perhaps even simply happy with the knowledge that she has helped to bring to others the joy of parenthood. Stefan and Nadia are, Keane could add, more typical than Bill and Bridget, John and Lorelei, or the Malahoffs.

In *The Surrogate Mother* Keane gave an account of his first nine cases. If we take this as a sample, then the cases of Bill and Bridget and of John and Lorelei were the two most tangled of these nine. Even so, one of these two had a happy ending. So would it have been right to prevent eight couples having the child they wanted, just in order to save John and Lorelei's disappointment?

In any case, Keane believes that the problems of his early cases could be avoided by changing the law so as to make surrogacy contracts enforceable, to legalize payment of a fee to a surrogate, and to enable the State to regulate surrogacy in roughly the same way as it now regulates adoption.

Let us consider first the problem of enforcing surrogacy contracts. Keane says that at present 'the practical reality' is that 'any and all contracts between adoptive couples and others wanting children, and their mothers are unenforceable'. Not surprisingly, there is little legal precedent in this area. The major case is a British one, which came to court in 1978. A professional man and a woman with whom he was living made an agreement with a prostitute that, in return for a fee; she would be artificially inseminated with the man's sperm, and would hand over the resulting child to the couple. When the child was born the mother refused to give up custody, despite the couple's offer to raise the fee very considerably. The dispute was taken to the Family Division of the High Court, where the judge ruled that the agreement was a contract for the sale of a child, and hence 'pernicious' and unenforceable. The prostitute kept her child.

It seems very likely that most courts in Britain and in Commonwealth countries like Australia would come to the same decision in any future similar cases. American courts are less predictable but Keane, as we have seen, is not optimistic about obtaining a different decision. Hence he would like legislation making such contracts enforceable at law. But how is this to be done?

Normally, contract law has at its disposal two 'remedies', one of which can be brought to bear on anyone in breach of a contract. If surrogacy contracts were to be made legally enforceable, they would have to be enforced by one or other of these two remedies. The first remedy is damages. This involves a court order to the defaulting party to pay a sum of money to the other party to the contract. Awarding damages in the case of a surrogate motherhood contract, however, will not help much. The couple will be wanting 'their' baby, not a sum of money, even if the defaulting surrogate were able to pay. Usually she won't be. Most paid surrogates will come from low-income groups and will be employed by members of high-income groups. Bearing children is not many women's idea of an easy time, and if it were not done from love or genuine altruism (in which case the matter would not be likely to come to court at all) the spur of economic necessity would need to be fairly deeply embedded. So in most cases the surrogate would not pay the damages awarded against her; and if she did, it would ruin her financially without giving much satisfaction to the couple who wanted the child.

The other remedy of contract law is called 'specific performance'. This means that the court compels the defaulting party to perform what he or she agreed to do under the contract. This is the form of enforcement that Keane would like to see applied to surrogacy contracts. Yet to apply it in this area could cause worse difficulties than it would solve. Suppose that a surrogate announced, soon after it was confirmed that she was pregnant, that the deal was off. She might say, for example, that she no longer felt she was psychologically adjusted to the idea of surrogate motherhood, and she wanted an abortion. Or she might say that she wished to bear the child but keep it herself. Could a court then step in and compel her to complete the contract—to bear the child and hand it over to the adopting couple? The compulsion involved would be of a uniquely odious form. The contract is not like an ordinary contract for services since its fulfilment involves physical invasion of the contractor's body. The surrogate could not, like any other contractor, walk out of the work-place. She is the work-place. Should she be taken into custody to prevent her obtaining an abortion? Should her baby be taken from her against her will, immediately after birth? Even in ordinary contracts for personal services the courts are unlikely to award specific performance, allowing only damages. In such cases judges have held that the analogy with slavery is too close. How much more so in the case of surrogacy.

In this kind of dispute, public opinion is clearly on the side of the surrogate mother. After asking people whether surrogate motherhood should be allowed, the Morgan Gallup poll went on to ask:

If the woman who gave birth to such a baby changed her mind, and wanted to *keep* the baby, *who* should have first claim on the baby—the couple whose fertilized egg was used, or the woman who gave birth to the child?

Australians favoured the woman who gave birth, by 35 per cent to 29 per cent, and Britons went still more clearly in that direction, with 50 per cent saying the woman who gave birth should have first claim on the baby, and only 19 per cent favouring the couple whose fertilized egg was used. When we keep in mind the fact that this question was about full surrogacy, and the surrogate's case for keeping the baby might well be thought to be stronger when she is also the genetic mother of the child, there can be little doubt that public opinion would not favour court orders compelling surrogates to give up the babies to whom they have given birth.

Despite the obvious difficulties, Keane thinks the law should be altered to make 'irrevocable' an agreement by the surrogate mother to release her parental rights to the adopting couple— even when the agreement is made before pregnancy begins. Such legislation is, in his view, 'absolutely essential' for the peace of mind of people pursuing surrogate parenting. He does not say how enforcement is to be carried out.

There are four ways in which the law could go on this issue. Firstly, it could, as Keane urges, give legal recognition and legal enforcement to surrogacy agreements. Secondly, it could go to the other extreme and ban surrogacy arrangements altogether, by making surrogacy a criminal act—as it may already be in those legal systems which prohibit unofficial adoptions, or (if a fee is involved) in legal systems which regard a surrogacy contract as a form of baby-selling. Thirdly, the law could take the middle way of declaring surrogacy contracts to be against public policy. This would mean that they were not enforceable at law, but it would not interfere with any private arrangements that people might like to make, at their own risk. Finally, some special means of regulating surrogacy might be devised.

In our view the law of contract is too blunt an instrument to enforce contracts for surrogate motherhood. In these situations neither the award of damages nor an order for specific perform-ance can do justice while satisfying anyone at all. For this reason we reject Keane's view.

Should we therefore go to the other extreme and ban surrogacy arrangements altogether? The trouble with this suggestion is that sometimes surrogate motherhood is motivated by genuine altruism, and occurs in a context which makes serious problems unlikely.

Consider, for instance, one final case from Keane's book: the story of George, Debbie, and Sue. Though the facts are related by Keane, he had nothing to do with their arrangement. He first heard from them when he appeared on a radio talk-show with Bill and Bridget. At that stage he had not arranged any surrogate pregnancies, but he had two couples looking for women willing to act as surrogates, and he was hopeful that the radio appearance might produce volunteers. Instead it produced a message that said: 'Call us. We've already done it.'

Indeed they had. Debbie was twenty-four and married to George, twenty-eight, when she became ill with severe stomach cramps. Rushed to hospital, she was found to have a womb so badly infected that the only thing the doctors could do was remove it. Debbie was devastated. She had always assumed she would have children. She tried adoption agencies, and was told that the waiting time was seven years. She was, she says, 'starting to go crackers'.

At this point Sue comes into the story. Sue was Debbie's closest friend, so close that Debbie's obvious distress at her inability to have a child had affected her as well. Suddenly Sue had the idea of being able to do something for her friend, to whom she felt she owed much. She offered to have a baby for them.

When Sue first mentioned the idea, George and Debbie thought it was a joke. Sue had thought only of having a baby by sexual intercourse with a man she knew. It was George who suggested that, if she was serious, they should use artificial insemination with his sperm. They read up on artificial insemination in, no kidding, the *Reader's Digest Family Health Guide* and decided that they could do it themselves. They did, with Debbie inserting George's semen into Sue's vagina by means of a syringe. Sue became pregnant on the first attempt, and nine months later handed Debbie and George a baby daughter, whom they subsequently legally adopted. Fourteen months after the birth, 'Auntie Sue' remained close to George and Debbie, and to the baby. As far as one can tell from Keane's account, everyone is happy with the way things have worked out.

Another instance of altruistic surrogacy, this time from France, produced a result that was, if possible, even more ideal. Magali Crozel was sterile. Her twin sister, Christine, offered to have a baby for her. After artificial insemination by Magali's husband, Christine duly gave birth to a son. Because Magali and Christine are identical twins, the boy was genetically indistinguishable from a child that Magali might have had, if she had not been sterile.

Should the law be changed so as to make criminals of people who act like George, Debbie, and Sue, or like Magali Crozel and her sister? In our view it should not be. These people may have acted unconventionally, but their motives were laudable, and there is nothing in what they did that threatens the fabric of our society or any individual members of it. Perhaps not every woman would want to act as Sue and Christine did; but we can see no basis for criminal sanctions against those who do. Of course, even in the best of circumstances things can go wrong. Things are markedly less likely to go wrong, however, when people are motivated by love and kindness, and act without demanding a reward.

Problems arise once money enters into the arrangement. The possibilities of exploitation are everywhere. Surrogates may extort money from couples desperate to have a child, as Diane extorted money from Bill and Bridget. Conversely, the use of a surrogate might become the hallmark of the idle rich, with the surrogate ousting the butler and the housemaid as a status symbol. This might of course be defended on the grounds that it would provide employment, but it runs strongly against the trend towards a society with fewer differences in class and status.

A child born of a volunteer surrogate mother might well feel, especially if it continued to have a loving relationship with the surrogate after its adoption, that it was more loved than a child who was borne for profit. Similarly a volunteer surrogate who performed her role out of love—whether to help a friend or as an expression of some more distant form of altruism—would be less likely to suffer violence to her emotions than one who made a profession of dissociating gestation from nurture. To prevent the expression of human altruism, where that altruism could be harnessed to the increase of human happiness, just because of the abuses that would occur where profit and not love became the motive, would be to throw the baby out with the bath water.

So far we have argued against making surrogacy contracts enforceable at law, but also against prohibiting them altogether. What then of the third possibility: permitting surrogacy arrangements, but refusing to allow the law to enforce them?

The objection to this 'hands off' approach by the law is that once surrogacy is allowed, some people will be ready to pay for it if they cannot find volunteers—and Keane's experience suggests that many will not be able to find a volunteer. In these circumstances, the adoptive couple will be inadequately protected. They will put their money down, but find themselves with a worthless contract which the courts will refuse to enforce. Some surrogates will take the money and run—first to an abortionist. Others will gradually turn the screw on the adoptive couple as their longed-for baby comes closer to its time of delivery.

One could take the hard line and say that since paid surrogacy contracts are against public policy, people who choose to enter such arrangements in the full knowledge that they are unenforceable must take the risk of being exploited. But this seems excessively hard in view of the weak position in which childless couples may find themselves. Most countries now recognize the need for laws to protect consumers. Are not childless couples who make surrogacy arrangements also consumers? If so, do they not merit protection?

The difficulty is to provide protection for the adoptive couple without falling back on the draconian remedy of compelling the unwilling surrogate to hand over the baby she now wishes to keep. We would favour a system of regulations designed not to solve the problem of the surrogate mother who changes her mine—for there can be no satisfactory solution to that problem— but designed to avoid the occurrence of that very situation.

How might this be done? The regulations governing adoption in some countries might serve as a model. Just as private adoptions are illegal, so private surrogacy agreements would be illegal. All those wanting a surrogate, or wanting to be a surrogate, would have to contact a State Surrogacy Board. The Board could try to encourage volunteers motivated by a desire to help others. For reasons we gave when discussing the analogous case of the payment of donors of sperm and eggs, we think it would be best if the Board began by seeing whether the demand for surrogate mothers could be met by volunteers. Only if it was clear that it could not, would the Board set a fee, at a level regarded as fair to all parties. The Board would carefully screen all potential surrogates. Adoptive couples might also be screened, as ordinary adoptive couples now are—except that the criteria would not have to be so strict, for the supply of surrogate mothers would not be as rigidly limited as the supply of children available for adoption. No contracts could be signed, or fees paid, except through the Board.

This system would have several advantages. Since the screening of surrogates would not be done by couples clutching at any straw in order to have a chance of a child, the prospects of avoiding alcoholics and drug addicts would be high. While the Board would not attempt to enforce contracts against surrogate mothers, the Board's expert screening panels might, with practice, be able to avoid the kind of woman most likely to change her mind about giving up the baby, or to suffer psychologically from the experience. If financial incentives did turn out to be needed to ensure a sufficient supply of surrogate mothers, the Board could withhold the bulk of the payment until after the child was given to the adoptive parents. Because she was dealing with a State Board, rather than with private citizens, the surrogate need not fear that after handing over the baby she might not get paid at all. At the same time, since the Board would act as a buffer between the couple and the surrogate, it would make it much more difficult for the surrogate to extort additional money from the couple.

A Surrogacy Board might also grapple with the question of who should be eligible to apply for a surrogate. As we saw earlier, there is a gradation of need, from couples who have no possibility of a child without a surrogate, to couples who could have a child at varying degrees of risk to the woman's health, to couples for whom pregnancy would be an interference with the woman's career, and finally to couples for whom pregnancy would be merely an inconvenience. Regulated surrogacy might begin cautiously, the Board accepting only infertile couples or couples in which pregnancy would be extremely risky for the woman. If after a few years all went well and the supply of surrogates was adequate to cover the needs of these groups, the Board might relax the criteria. Separate waiting lists could be established for different groups, and while the costs of those with medical reasons for seeking surrogacy might be subsidized by State health funds, others would pay the full cost.

All these issues need careful thought; but it is too early to produce a detailed blueprint of how regulated surrogacy might work. In this area piecemeal social engineering is the way to make progress.

Partial surrogacy, at least, is here to stay. It does not require the intervention of a doctor. George, Debbie, and Sue managed artificial insemination on their own; and if that had failed, they could have followed the example of Abram, Sarai, and Hagar. Even if attempts to suppress partial surrogacy were justified— and we do not think they are—such attempts would merely drive it underground. We do not claim that a Surrogacy Board will bring about problem-free surrogacy, but we do think it has the capacity greatly to reduce the incidence of problems in this area. It is clearly preferable to unregulated surrogacy, whether legal or illegal, and also preferable to attempts to enforce contracts against surrogates. While a prohibition on private surrogacy arrangements will always be difficult to enforce, the availability of officially regulated surrogacy would eliminate most of the motivation for such private arrangements. Regulation is, therefore, preferable to any other alternative that has been proposed or that we are able to envisage.

Partial surrogacy or full surrogacy?

Our discussion has been based on partial surrogacy, because that is the only form of surrogacy of which anyone has any experience. Is there any relevant difference between the two which means that the conclusions we have reached should not be applied to full surrogacy?

One difference is that whereas partial surrogacy can be accomplished without medical expertise or hospital facilities, full surrogacy cannot be. It requires all the skill and equipment needed to bring IVF to a successful outcome. This means that whereas attempts to suppress partial surrogacy would, as we have just argued, merely drive it underground, full surrogacy could be stopped much more easily. But is there any reason why, if partial surrogacy is allowed to go ahead in the manner we suggested, full surrogacy should be prohibited?

Remember that we are not asking this question in a vacuum. For the reasons we have given, partial surrogacy seems certain to continue whether we like it or not. If full surrogacy were allowed, it would probably take the place of at least some of the partial surrogacy arrangements, rather than contribute to a larger overall number of surrogate births. Given this, we think that no attempt should be made to prohibit full surrogacy; for we think that full surrogacy, once perfected, would be preferable to partial surrogacy.

The basis for this preference is that with full surrogacy both the adopting parents are the genetic parents of the child they will bring up. This has advantages for the couple, the child, and the surrogate. For the couple, the child really is 'their child' in a way that it cannot be when partial surrogacy is used. For this reason most couples would want full surrogacy rather than partial surrogacy, if given the choice. And why should we deny them the choice?

Full surrogacy also avoids the possible future psychological problems of children who want to know more about their genetic mothers. In full surrogacy, the role of the surrogate mother can be regarded as a temporary intervention: something needed to take the embryo from the stage of fertilization to the point at which there is a baby capable of surviving outside the womb. This may not have any lasting effects on the child. Later in life, therefore, if the children initially feel uncomfortable about having had surrogate mothers, they can put the whole episode firmly in the past, and say that what they are *now* has not been affected by what happened then. The children of partial surrogacy know that the opposite is true: what happened then has left its permanent marks upon them. They cannot distance their present self from the surrogate who carried them, because they will always carry the characteristics they have inherited from the surrogates. In this respect the children of partial surrogacy may experience some of the anxiety about their genetic mothers that the children of artificial insemination may have about their genetic fathers. We discussed these problems in Chapter 3, and did not find that they amounted to an overwhelming objection to the use of donor sperm or donor eggs. Similarly, they do not amount to an overwhelming objection to partial surrogacy; but if they can be avoided by the use of full surrogacy, so much the better.

Finally, and for the same reason, full surrogacy is likely to be easier for the surrogate mother. Mothers who give up children for adoption often say that they find it very distressing not to know what has happened to their child. Is she alive or dead? Does he look like me? Some of these mothers say that they search among crowds of schoolchildren of the right age, looking for a face they might recognize. Partial surrogate mothers may well feel as these mothers do; but full surrogate mothers would feel less of a bond between themselves and the child they bore. A full surrogate mother would be more like a wet nurse or a nanny, someone who was close to the child for a time and so might well take an interest in its future, without ever feeling that the child was in any way *her* child. The full surrogate mother could never expect to recognize her child's face in a crowd by its resemblance to her own; presumably she would be less likely to search for it.

Conclusions

To conclude this chapter, we shall sum up our argument for permitting full surrogate motherhood, on a strictly regulated basis.

We began with some reasons why people might want surrogacy. We saw that in some cases surrogate motherhood might be the only way in which a couple could have a child. We then looked at objections to surrogacy, and illustrated them with problems arising from actual cases of partial surrogacy. These problems were very serious, but they did not seem to justify making partial surrogacy a criminal offence. Taking that course met with two powerful objections: it would make criminals of people motivated by love or altruism and who, in the view of many reasonable observers, would have done nothing wrong; and it would be more likely to drive partial surrogacy underground than to stop the practice altogether. Instead of prohibition, therefore, we suggested regulation of partial surrogacy by a Surrogacy Board which would be able to avoid many of the problems that have occurred with unregulated partial surrogacy. We then compared partial surrogacy and full surrogacy, and found that full surrogacy had advantages for the couple, the child, and the surrogate mother. Since the availability of full surrogacy seems certain to mean fewer partial surrogacies rather than a greater total number of surrogate arrangements, this comparison led us straight to the conclusion that the Surrogacy Board should permit full surrogate motherhood.

5 ECTOGENESIS

The prospects

On 4 January 1981, Faye Bland went into premature labour. Only six and a half months pregnant, she fully expected to lose the baby. She was rushed into the Queen Victoria Medical Centre, where doctors attempted to stop the labour. Despite their efforts, some thirty hours later Kim Bland was born. He was alive but tiny, weighing only 470 grams, or just over 1 lb. in imperial weights. Nevertheless the doctors used all the modern technology of neonatal intensive care units. He was fed through a tube, and kept warm in a humidicrib. He did not die. At first he lost weight, dropping to a mere 420 grams; but then he started gaining. Kim had his problems. When he weighed 1,130 grams (2½ lb.) he had a hernia operation. At six weeks of age, he had a leg fracture due to calcium deficiency. But he continued to grow, came out of the humidicrib, and could be fed from a bottle. A year later Kim came back to the hospital for birthday celebrations. He was the smallest baby to have survived at the Queen Victoria Medical Centre, and one of the smallest anywhere in the world. Though extreme prematurity often leads to some form of handicap, Kim was entirely normal.

Ten years ago, a baby like Kim Bland would have had no chance of survival. Doctors' efforts were concentrated on trying to save babies weighing around 1,500 grams: those weighing under 1,000 grams were allowed to die because nothing much could be done for them. Now it is common for babies born three or even three and a half months premature to be pulled through the difficult early stages. If present trends continue, there seems little doubt that in another ten years time, there will be nothing remarkable about the survival of a baby weighing 470 grams, and even smaller and more premature babies, now regarded as impossible to save, will be surviving.

Whether this investment in highly sophisticated and extremely expensive medical technology is a good thing is not the point at issue here. Some oppose it, on the grounds that medical resources could be better invested elsewhere; others say that the number of infants surviving but severely handicapped is too high a price to pay in terms of human suffering. We shall not enter into this difficult discussion now. Our reference to these developments is simply intended to make the point that the human foetus no longer needs to be in a human womb for anything like the normal nine months. Ectogenesis—the growth and development of a being outside its mother's womb during the period when it would normally be inside the womb—is already a partial reality. Will complete ectogenesis also become a reality in the near future? And if it does, what should be done about it?

The period in which it is necessary for the human foetus to be in its mother's womb is shrinking from both sides. Conception can occur in the laboratory, and the newly created embryo can be kept alive for two or three days, while the original single cell splits, and each cell splits again, and again, until the embryo consists of sixteen cells. Then, under present procedures, it is essential to place the embryo in the womb if a pregnancy is to be achieved. According to the published literature, there has not been a pregnancy resulting from implantation of an embryo after more than three days *in vitro*, or of more than thirty-two cells. While they have not been successfully implanted, however, embryos have been kept alive for longer periods. In 1975, Robert Edwards kept three surplus embryos alive, instead of dissecting them for microscopic examination, as he had done with others. One of them continued to grow for nine days before Edwards, fearful that it would die unexamined, prepared it for dissection. Edwards describes it in these terms:

The embryo was still a speck, only just visible in our culture dish, but for me it represented the crucial stages of human embryology, the actual moments when the foundations are being laid for the formation of the body's organs. Cells and tissues grew and moved, assuming new forms in readiness for the moment when the embryo would begin to take a recognizable shape. Normally, of course, the embryo would be developing in this way inside its mother's womb, but I was privileged to watch it in our culture dish with all its promise of future growth.

That particular embryo might have lived even longer than nine days if Edwards had not decided to dissect it. Yet Edwards himself has not been able to repeat his early success in keeping an embryo alive for so long. Another Cambridge physiologist, however, has had more success with other species. Dennis New has been able to keep mouse and rat embryos alive for about two weeks. When allowance is made for the normal duration of pregnancy, this is roughly equivalent to four weeks of human embryonic life. By this stage the mouse and rat embryos have formed all their organs and the placenta.

Thus the present gap of a little over five months during which the natural womb is absolutely essential will certainly be reduced, and may end up being eliminated altogether. This will occur almost by accident, because the ability to keep the immature foetus alive outside the womb will not be developed by researchers deliberately seeking to make ectogenesis possible, but rather by doctors attempting to save the lives of premature babies. At the other end, it is hard to imagine that researchers investigating early embryo development will not, sooner or later, discover the defect in the laboratory environment which makes embryos cease to grow beyond a certain stage. Why should the replication of the condition of the womb be an insoluble mystery, when the problem of replicating the conditions necessary for conception have been solved?

Having stumbled on ectogenesis in this manner, we shall then have to decide whether to make use of the possibility thus created.

The case for ectogenesis

The medical grounds

Medically speaking, ectogenesis offers an alternative to surrogate motherhood for women who are incapable of pregnancy, or for whom pregnancy is not recommended on medical grounds. As we saw in our discussion of surrogate motherhood, the most likely cases are women who have had a hysterectomy, or women with a health problem which could be worsened by pregnancy. Such women would still provide fertile eggs. These could be obtained by laparoscopy, fertilized *in vitro* with their partner's sperm, and the embryo would then continue to grow 'in the test-tube'—actually in some much more complicated kind of artificial womb—until it was old enough to be 'born', presumably first into a humidicrib and only later into the normal environment.

The medical case for ectogenesis, then, would consist of the medical case for surrogate motherhood, coupled with the claim that ectogenesis should be chosen in preference to surrogacy. The reason for this preference might be one of the objections to surrogate motherhood we have already discussed. If, for instance, early experience with surrogacy showed that surrogate mothers could not be relied upon to give up to its genetic parents the child they had carried, ectogenesis might be thought better than a battle over custody. Evidence that surrogate mothers frequently smoked, or took alcohol or drugs that caused harm to the baby might be another reason for preferring the strictly controlled artificial environment. It might be that in a voluntary system there would be a shortage of women willing to be surrogates. It might be, in a country that opted for a market system, that the cost of employing a surrogate is too high, and ectogenesis—once it becomes a standard procedure—is a more economical alternative.

The end of abortion?

Odd as it may seem, ectogenesis conceivably could win the support of right-to-life organizations and others opposed to abortion. Those who take this view are opposed, of course, to any experiments on the human embryo which carry a risk of its death; but efforts to save the lives of premature babies are not experiments in this sense. The techniques used may be experimental, but they will be acceptable as long as they give the baby a greater chance of life than it would otherwise have. Thus those who believe that the embryo is a human being from the moment of conception must support medical developments which are extending the period during which a natural womb is not required. Since for those who take this view there is no point, before conception, at which the embryo lacks a right to life, there is no point at which this process of extension should stop. They should support its extension to all cases of spontaneous—that is, not deliberately induced—abortion, no matter how soon after conception the spontaneous abortion should occur.

And what of deliberately induced abortions? Eetogenesis could at some future time make right-to-life organizations drop their objections to abortion; for it is only our inability to keep early foetuses alive that makes abortion synonymous with the violation of any right to life which the foetus may have. If we could keep a foetus alive, outside the body, abortions could be done using techniques that would not harm the foetuses, and the foetuses, or new-born babies as they would then be, could be adopted—if there were enough willing couples. Abortions would in effect become early births, and the destruction of the unborn would cease.

Would those who now argue for the permissibility of abortion object to this development? If the feminist argument for abortion takes its stand on the right of women to control their own bodies, feminists at least should not object. Freedom to choose what is to happen to one's body is one thing; freedom to insist on the death of a being that is capable of living outside one's body is another. At present these two are inextricably linked, and so the woman's freedom to choose conflicts head-on with the alleged right to life of the foetus. When ectogenesis becomes possible these two issues will break apart, and women will choose to terminate their pregnancies without thereby choosing the inevitable death of the foetus they are carrying. Pro-choice feminists and pro-foetus right-to-lifers can then embrace in happy harmony.

Some who now defend abortion might still object that the woman has a right to decide whether her embryo lives or dies. She may not wish to keep it, and yet she may not like the idea of it being handed over to another couple. So should she not have the right to have it aborted in a manner that ensures its death? But this is a very different argument from the usual pro-choice argument for abortion. It could only be accepted if the claim that the foetus has a right to life had been disproved, and even then it is difficult to see why a healthy foetus should die if there is someone who wishes to adopt it and will give it the opportunity of a worthwhile life. We do not now allow a mother to kill her new-born baby because she does not wish either to keep it or to hand it over for adoption. Unless we were to change our mind about this, it is difficult to see why we should give this right to a woman in respect of a foetus she is carrying, if her desire to be rid of the foetus can be fully satisfied without threatening the life of the foetus.

Those opposed to abortion thus ought to welcome the development of ectogenesis, at least in so far as it can be developed without deliberately risking the lives of embryos in experimental work. Feminists, too, should welcome it for the simple reason that it promises to defuse the whole abortion issue, and thus end the threat that opponents of abortion will one day succeed in their efforts to deny women the freedom to control their own reproductive organs.

Reproductive equality?

In *The Dialectic of Sex*, one of the seminal works of the modern feminist movement, Shulamith Firestone argues that the ultimate cause of inequality between the sexes is simply the natural reproductive difference between males and females. The biological family forms a basic reproductive unit, but within this unit the division of biological labour is fundamentally unequal. Women must go through pregnancy and childbirth, breast-feeding, and caring for the infants. All this restricts their ability to be self-sufficient, and makes them dependent on males for physical survival. Venturing further still, Firestone suggests that this initial division of reproductive labour led directly to the general division of labour between males and females, and in turn is at the root of further divisions into economic and cultural classes. Thus she claims to have taken Marx's analysis of the economic division of labour back one step further, to its roots in the biological division of the sexes.

Some feminists are understandably reluctant to accept Firestone's view. If the basic cause of women's inequality is the natural method of continuing our species, the prospects of achieving equality look dim. Most feminists are happier attributing female inequality to upbringing and indoctrination, leaving biological explanations to those who say that male supremacy is natural and unchanging. Firestone, however, has the boldness to offer a biological reason for female inequality, and then urge us to do something about it. Her solution is ectogenesis:

I submit, then, that the first demand for any alternative system must be:
1) *The freeing of women from the tyranny of their reproductive biology by every*

means available, and the diffusion of the childbearing and childrearing role to the
society as a whole, men as well as women.

Firestone makes it clear that she is not talking simply about
better day-care centres, not even 'twenty-four-hour child-care
centres staffed by men as well as women'. Such proposals she
describes as 'timid'. Rather she looks to the 'potentials of modern
embryology, possibilities still so frightening that they are seldom
discussed seriously'.

Why do we seldom take these possibilities seriously? One
response might be that at the time Firestone was writing, several
years before the first successful human fertilization outside the
body, ectogenesis seemed too remote to be worth discussion.
Firestone, however, has a deeper explanation. Science is in male
hands. Just as, in the view of many feminists, the development of
a male oral contraceptive has been slowed by male reluctance to
share the risks and responsibilities of contraception, so in
Firestone's view research into developing new methods of
reproduction has been impeded by reluctance to accept new
possibilities that could upset the traditional male-dominated
family structure. In support of this thesis she points to a fact that
we have already noted: any progress toward ectogenesis that has
already occurred has not been aimed deliberately at that goal as
something itself desirable because of the new options it would
create for women. It has been justified on the grounds that it may
save babies born prematurely. (Firestone might now add that, at
the other end of pregnancy, the development of external
fertilization had to be justified on the grounds that it will enable
infertile women to fulfil the desire to bear children!)

Ectogenesis, then, can be supported on the ground that it
would make a fundamental contribution toward sexual equality.
Feminists who accept this argument will wish to see research into
the development of complete ectogenesis pushed ahead with
all due speed.

Better adjusted children?

For the sake of completeness, we mention another argument
advanced, almost incidentally, by Firestone in her defence of
ectogenesis. As ectogenesis liberates women from the burden of
pregnancy and childbirth, so too, according to Firestone, it would

liberate children from the burden of possessive mothering. In discussing the kind of household unit she would like to see in the future, when there would be full equality between the sexes, she says:

we must be aware that as long as we use natural childbirth methods, the 'household' could never be a totally liberating social form. A mother who undergoes a nine-month pregnancy is likely to feel that the product of all that pain and discomfort 'belongs' to her ('To think of what I went through to have you!'). But we want to destroy this possessiveness along with its cultural reinforcements so that . . . children will be loved for their own sake.

Firestone's claim is that children nurtured from conception outside the body will have a healthier relationship with their mother than normal children. This assertion makes, as we shall see, an interesting contrast to one common objection to ectogenesis. It is now time to turn to this and other objections.

The embryo as a source of spare parts

The final argument for ectogenesis will enthuse some and be utterly repugnant to others. It is that embryos could be kept alive as a source of tissues and organs that could be of great benefit to more mature humans.

Modern medicine uses tissue and organ transplants for a wide variety of purposes. Kidney transplants are obviously to be preferred to lifelong dialysis in patients with kidney disease. Bone marrow grafts can be life-saving in patients being treated for leukaemia. Cornea transplants have restored the sight of many people with clouded vision. More experimentally, the transplantation of cells from the pancreas is being tried as a means of overcoming diabetes, and there is even talk of the transplantation of brain tissue to overcome brain damage, and of nerve tissue to repair the nervous systems of those with spinal injuries.

There are at present two major limitations on the use of tissue and organ transplants. The first is the problem of rejection. Unless the donor is a close relative, the probability is great that the body of the recipient will attack the donated tissue as if it were a foreign body. Heavy doses of drugs can sometimes suppress this reaction, but they have their own side-effects. The risk of rejection varies with the particular tissue being used; in some cases the only way to overcome rejection is for the donated tissue to come from an identical twin, but of course identical twins are not often available.

The second problem is that it is difficult to obtain sufficient organs for transplantation. With something like blood, or skin, which will regenerate, it is easy enough to find a donor; but to give up a kidney is a serious matter for a living donor, while brain or nerve tissue, or a liver or a pancreas, could be taken only from a corpse.

The use of embryos could overcome these limitations. If the embryos were specially grown for the purpose, there would be no shortage of tissue. As for rejection, there is some evidence that embryonic tissue is not as likely to be rejected as adult tissue. But there is also a much more dramatic prospect. As Robert Edwards pointed out at a meeting at Bourn Hall, Cambridge, in 1981, the embryos could be genetically 'tailor-made' for the individuals who needed them, so that rejection would not occur. One way of doing this would be by cloning, a technique we shall describe in a later chapter. So far as our present topic is concerned, the essential point is that cloning could produce individuals genetically identical to the person whose cells are used to start the clone. For the purposes of transplanting, a clone would be as good as an identical twin.

It might be thought that embryos are too tiny to produce useful amounts of tissue, or organs of the size needed by an adult. Provided the embryos can be kept alive until they have started to form the necessary tissue or organs, however, it might be possible to remove the tissue or organs, and keep them alive in a culture. Given the right nutrients the organs would grow very rapidly to normal adult size. This prospect is certainly still some years distant, but it is not impossible that we might one day grow embryos so as to save the lives of those with diseased kidneys, livers, or hearts, to enable diabetics to produce their own insulin, and to provide nerve tissue that could make paraplegics walk again.

This would be partial, not complete ectogenesis, since obviously the embryo is not brought through to a time when it can survive on its own. Its survival is not the aim of the procedure: the survival of others is.

Objections to Ectogenesis

The ectogenetic child

Suppose that we develop the technical ability to keep an embryo alive and growing outside its mother's womb. How could there be any guarantee that the subsequent child would develop normally? Might there not be something, whether chemical or emotional, which is transmitted from the mother to her child during pregnancy, and which we are unable to detect? Without this element, mightn't the child be permanently disadvantaged, physically or mentally?

Given our lack of complete knowledge of the conditions needed for fully normal, well-adjusted children, any attempt to nurture a child entirely outside the womb would be experimentation with human life. It would be an especially reckless form of experimentation because it would be several years before it could be established if the children of ectogenesis were normal in their emotional and mental development; meanwhile several thousand ectogenetic children might have been brought into existence, all destined for a deprived human life. Therefore, those who urge this objection will say, ectogenesis should be totally prohibited.

The ectogenetic mother

Shulamith Firestone saw the special mother–child relationship as an aspect of female inequality, and therefore something to be done away with if at all possible. More traditionally minded people might object to ectogenesis on the grounds that mothers are better, more caring parents precisely because they have carried the child in so intimate a manner. The bonding thus begun already in pregnancy continues after birth, these people would say, and is desirable not only from the point of view of the child, but also from the point of view of the woman, for whom the experience is more emotionally fulfilling than any other.

Viewed through traditional eyes, a woman who could become pregnant but chose ectogenesis would be shirking her obligations as a mother and denying her essential identity as a woman. Granted, pregnancy can be uncomfortable and childbirth can be painful, but they are part of the collective experience of womanhood and no woman can avoid them without feeling a lack of fulfilment, with subsequent damage to her feminine psyche.

Unnaturalness

This objection should by now be familiar. Those who consider *in vitro* fertilization 'unnatural' will certainly consider ectogenesis still more so. Undoubtedly it *is* still more unnatural, in the sense in which anything that is the result of the application of human intelligence to the task of altering our basic biological condition is 'unnatural'. In that sense, even surrogate motherhood is closer to our natural condition than ectogenesis, for surrogate motherhood at least uses all the normal biological resources of the female body.

Approaching Brave New World

Here is another familiar objection. If the term 'test-tube babies' was instantly applied to *in vitro* fertilization, how much more appropriate it is for the embryo developing entirely outside the body. In fact ectogenesis will certainly not take place in anything as simple as a test-tube, but the parallel is nevertheless far closer than it was in the simpler case of IVF. Ectogenesis would make it technically possible to mass-produce babies in the manner Aldous Huxley describes in *Brave New World*. For this reason, some will say, we should not move toward ectogenesis. There are some forms of knowledge it would be better not to have.

Farming human beings

Finally there is the objection to the use of the embryo as a means of growing organs as spare parts. For anyone who holds that from the moment of conception there is a human being, with the same right to life as any other human being, the suggestion that we grow embryos for spare parts amounts to a proposal to farm—and subsequently slaughter—human beings. From this perspective it would be the most grotesque violation of human rights imaginable, a form of slavery in which even the life of the slave is not spared. It would be the deliberate and institutionalized violation of the most fundamental of all human rights.

142   *Ectogenesis*

Discussion

We listed five reasons for going ahead with ectogenesis: to help couples who cannot otherwise have a child, except by the use of a surrogate, where for some reason ectogenesis is preferred to surrogacy; to create a source of spare parts needed to replace diseased organs; to eliminate the wastage of embryonic life now caused by abortion; to eliminate the present inequality in the division of reproductive labour; and to reduce the possessiveness of natural mothers. In the absence of any decisive objections to ectogenesis, any one of the first four reasons would be sufficient to justify the procedure. None of them is altogether negligible. Helping infertile couples is, in itself, a good thing. So is—even more obviously—saving the lives of those who would otherwise die from a deteriorating heart or kidney. While there is debate over the status of embryonic life, who would deny the value of a procedure that would allow women complete control over their reproduction and at the same time end the present waiting list for adoption?

Rather more radical is the idea that there is positive value in the elimination of as much as possible of the differences between the reproductive roles of males and females. Not everyone will agree that equality should go this far. But Firestone's suggestion might receive wider acceptance if the emphasis were placed more on the enhancement of individual freedom that ectogenesis would bring. Women would not, after all, be compelled to use the new method; all it would do is provide them with a new option. If they wished to avoid pregnancy and childbirth while still having a child of their own, they could; if they preferred the traditional experience, they could of course go through with it all in the traditional manner. Since freedom is almost universally recognized as a good, when Firestone's argument is put in this manner, it too must be generally agreed to carry at least some weight.

We shall not offer any opinion on the fifth reason for ectogenesis—Firestone's claim that the children of ectogenesis would be better adjusted. Whether this would be so is, in our view, impossible to decide before such children exist. Nevertheless, the first four reasons are ample to make out a valid case for ectogenesis. The initial task of our discussion will therefore be to consider whether any of the objections offered—or the sum of them all—amounts to a sufficiently serious reason to outweigh the case in favour.

Let us first consider complete ectogenesis, and later deal separately with the proposal to use the embryo as a source of spare parts.

In our view three of the four objections to complete ectogenesis can readily be dismissed. What we have said earlier about the term 'unnatural' can be applied here. There is no appropriate sense of 'unnatural' in which respirators for premature babies are natural but ectogenesis is unnatural; yet the opponents of ectogenesis do not wish to oppose respirators. In any case, as we have already seen, there is no valid argument from 'unnatural' to 'wrong'. Similarly, while ectogenesis obviously does bring us closer to 'Brave New World' in one respect, as we pointed out before, the reasons we object to the society Huxley has described have a lot to do with the political and moral ideals of that society, and relatively little to do with its technical capabilities.

For a different reason, we would also dismiss the objection that ectogenesis is undesirable from the standpoint of the ectogenetic mother. We dismiss this objection not because we deny the value, for many women, of the experience of pregnancy and childbirth 'the natural way'. Obviously some radical feminists would deny this value. Firestone, for example, flatly states: 'Pregnancy is *barbaric*' and quotes a description of childbirth as 'like shitting a pumpkin'. It is not necessary for us to take sides on this issue, however, because women are responsible agents capable of choosing for themselves whether to have the experience in question. It would be an act of extraordinary paternalism—never mind about male chauvinism—for a government to tell women that because it knew that pregnancy was good for them, it would not allow the development of alternative means of producing babies.

There may be situations where the case for protecting people against their own folly is so strong that paternalism is justified—compulsory use of helmets by motorcyclists might be an example—but this is surely not one of them. The value that would be enforced—that is, the value of going through the traditional experience of pregnancy and childbirth—is nowhere near as clear-cut as the value of avoiding the head injuries that are more likely to be suffered by motorcyclists without helmets. While no one denies the value of avoiding such injuries, some people do question, and not unreasonably, the value of pregnancy. Paternalism to enforce so contested a value cannot be justified. Women should be allowed to decide what they value and act accordingly. If, as the objection claims, pregnancy and childbirth are such rewarding experiences for women, those in favour of the traditional method should have nothing to fear: word will soon spread, and ectogenesis will exist only as the last resort of the otherwise infertile woman.

The most likely situation, in fact, is that ectogenesis, like most technologies, will suit some women and not others. Since this particular technology will—with one possible exception to be considered in a moment—have no harmful effects on those who do not choose to use it, the fact that it will not suit everyone is no reason why those who prefer it should not have access to it.

But is it true that ectogenesis will have no harmful effects on those who do not choose to use it? What about the ectogenetic child? This brings us to the most serious difficulty in the way of going ahead with ectogenesis: will the ectogenetic child develop normally?

We saw earlier that the same objection was made to *in vitro* fertilization, when the technique was in its experimental stage. Fears that IVF will lead to a high incidence of abnormal babies have now been set at rest; but this alone does not prove that scientists were justified in taking the risk. Winning a gamble does not always show that taking the gamble was wise in the first place. The only thing that can justify the decision is a careful assessment of the risks as they appeared at the time, leading to the conclusion that the knowledge then available provided a sufficient basis for the belief that the offspring of IVF would not have significantly more defects than children conceived by the usual method.

The same standard should apply to ectogenesis. To meet it may be more difficult than in the case of IVF. *In vitro* fertilization in humans was based on wide experience of the commercial use of the technique in farm animals, particularly cattle. The resulting offspring had been normal; and while species do vary, there was no reason to think humans and cattle would be different in this respect. Further evidence was provided by laboratory observation of human embryos fertilized outside the body and kept alive in culture for a day or two. Several scientists regarded this as sufficient basis for going ahead with IVF in humans, although they were criticized for so doing by bioethicists like Leon Kass and Paul Ramsey. The problem with ectogenesis is that any work done with non-human animals will be less readily applicable to humans than it was in the case of IVF. This is because with ectogenesis the worries would be about whether the baby would turn out normal in a mental and psychological sense—and here the data to be obtained from cattle breeding would not help much. Laboratory studies would also be of little use, since it is hard to imagine how anything could be discovered without letting the experiment run its full course, thus producing a child who might very well turn out abnormal. But if it is unethical to attempt ectogenesis in humans until we have a reasonable assurance that it is safe, and we can have no reasonable assurance that it is safe until it has been carried out, we seem to be in a classic 'catch 22' situation. Work on ectogenesis will remain forever unjustifiable.

Is there any way of breaking through this circle? We can see only one possibility. We mentioned earlier that ectogenesis might arise almost by accident. If we continue to push back the age at which premature babies can be saved, we shall eventually reach the point at which the human embryo produced through IVF can be kept alive without ever putting it inside a human body. We will then have achieved ectogenesis. If this process is a gradual one, and we constantly monitor the results of saving these earlier and earlier premature babies, there will not have been any unethical experimentation with human lives. At every stage we will have been doing our best to save the lives of premature babies. The work will have been medical, for the benefit of the patient, rather than scientific, to increase our knowledge—although of course this kind of classification is very rough and the use of new medical techniques often has both a medical and a scientific element.

The essential point is to work up to ectogenesis very gradually. The first step would be for it to become quite routine to save babies born at twenty-four weeks and weighing around 500 grams. We have not quite reached this point, but we are close to it. The next step would be to test these very premature babies at a stage when their mental and psychological development can be measured. This might require waiting as many as six years. Then, if these tests showed that the children had not been harmed by their experience, we could attempt to save even more premature babies. One complicating factor would be that premature babies have a higher rate of handicap than normal children, because a defective foetus is more likely to abort spontaneously, or be born prematurely, than a normal foetus. A higher rate of handicap among premature babies might therefore not indicate that premature birth itself did any harm to a normal baby, and would therefore not be a reason against ectogenesis. One would have to try to isolate the effect of prematurity from these other reasons for abnormality.

By this method we might reach ectogenesis in an ethical manner, although it would take many years. Ironically, some of the very people who oppose IVF—and would presumably oppose any direct attempt at ectogenesis—because of the risk involved, would think that the method we have outlined above is *too* slow and cautious. This is because they would regard every premature baby as a human being, with the same entitlement to have a major effort made to save its life as any other human being would have. Degree of prematurity or risk of major handicap would not be factors they would accept as counting against the obligation to try to save life. Therefore they would reject our suggestion that before trying to save a 400 gram baby, we should have some evidence that saving 500 gram babies does not lead to a tragically high rate of handicap, with the result that it produces more misery all round than there would have been if these babies had not been saved. They would not regard quality of life considerations as a reason for not saving human life, if we have the technical means of saving it.

For reasons given in our earlier discussion of the moral status of the embryo, we do not accept this view of the sanctity of every human life, irrespective of its quality. Hence our more cautious approach to saving premature infants, and to complete ectogenesis. We have mentioned the alternative view only in order to show that applying a 'right to life' ethic in this area would, paradoxi-cally, speed up development in the direction of ectogenesis. The overall conclusion is that whatever ethical stance we take, eventually there is going to be enough evidence of the safety of the procedures involved to justify the decision to go ahead with ectogenesis. Thus this final and most serious of the objections to ectogenesis is also not conclusive. It is sufficient to put ectogenesis out of bounds for the immediate future, but in twenty years the situation may be very different.

It remains only for us to consider partial ectogenesis—the proposal to use embryos as a source of organs for transplant surgery. There are internationally accepted guide-lines governing the use of human spare parts in transplant surgery. The recognized criterion for the permissibility of transplants of non-regenerative and unpaired body parts is brain death. The total absence of brain function indicates that vital organs may be taken from the body.

In Chapter 3, in discussing the moral status of the embryo, we suggested that if the medical profession and the community as a whole recognize, as they do, a body's lack of functional brain as a sufficient condition for utilizing transplantable material, then this condition is clearly applicable to, and met by, the early embryo. That is to say, the medical profession's own criterion, logically applied, should legitimate the surgical use of embryonic material for culture and subsequent use as replacement organs, or for research, up to the point at which the brain begins to function.

Of course, it might be objected that an embryo which has not developed a brain has the potential to do so, whereas a brain-dead individual does not have the potential to have a functioning brain. We have already argued against such arguments from potential, in Chapter 3. The potential of the embryo does not distinguish it from the egg and sperm, when considered jointly.

We are fortified in our view by the fact that until the brain and nervous system develop, there is no possibility of feeling pain—no more possibility, and indeed less, than brain-dead individuals who are at present our only source of parts for transplant surgery. Would those who rally to insist upon the inviolability of non-sentient embryos be equally opposed to the use of brain-dead individuals for transplant surgery, thus putting an end to that life-saving therapy? For that matter, would they be equally opposed to the use of highly sentient animals—like dogs or baboons—which, though they feel pain as acutely as we, are freely used in scientific research or for spare parts? In our view, this is a more serious moral issue, yet many people appear to be more strongly opposed to the use of non-sentient embryos.

We want to be perfectly clear about how far this can be taken. If there is any suspicion that an embryo has developed the rudiments of a brain, or that it has become sentient, then it is too late for it to be used for any sort of transplant surgery or research. There must always be a safety margin. No being—of any species— deserves to have gratuitous pain inflicted upon it.

There is one ambiguity about our conclusion that needs to be cleared up. What if an embryo were kept alive beyond the point at which it might normally experience pain; but before this point had been reached, an operation was performed which destroyed the parts of the brain involved in conscious experience? The embryo could then be grown indefinitely without ever being aware of anything. Would this put it in the same ethical category as the early embryo that is incapable of conscious experience?

Here we have a prospect that almost everyone will find repellent: the prospect of growing embryos until they resemble normal babies, but with their brains deliberately damaged so that they are in a permanent coma. On the other hand, if it is permissible to grow an embryo for two or three weeks and then terminate its existence, why should it not be permissible to keep it alive while eliminating its capacity for consciousness? To the embryo itself it can make no difference—either way it never will become a being with any feelings. So should we put aside our emotional reaction to the idea, and treat the two cases alike?

On this proposal we would emphatically urge caution. If all feelings are put aside, it has to be granted that there is no difference in the moral status of the pre-sentient embryo and the embryo with its capacity for sentience removed. Yet our feelings are not as easy to put aside as such blithe hypothetical statements make it appear. Throughout this book we have rejected the arguments of those who claim that new developments in reproduction would damage 'the moral fabric of our society', where this vague expression stands for some nebulous under-standing about marriage or procreation. The proposal we are now considering, however, could do violence to basic attitudes that are more specific and also more fundamental. For reasons that are to be found in our evolution as mammals bearing infants dependent on their parents for a long period, our attitude of care and protection to infants goes very deep. For normal adults, these feelings are an instinctive response to the appearance and behaviour of a baby. (They are not evoked by the sight of an embryo — again, for obvious evolutionary reasons.) These feelings are likely to be evoked by the sight of a new-born baby even if we know the baby is incapable of feeling anything. Sometimes, of course, we have to override these feelings, and apply our knowledge in the best interests of all concerned. For example, when a baby is born with a grave defect that will mean that its life is going to be miserable and brief, we may decide to allow it to die, rather than continue a life that can only bring suffering. To face these situations when they are forced upon us is one thing; to set up such conflicts deliberately is another. For the sake of the welfare of all our children, the basic attitude of care and protection for infants is one we must not imperil. We think this sufficient reason for rejecting, at least for the foreseeable future, the proposal to grow non-sentient embryos beyond the point at which they would normally have become sentient.

6 CLONING AND SEX SELECTION

In 1978 the respected New York publisher J. P. Lippincott announced a book of unusual interest: *In His Image*, by science writer David Rorvik. The subtitle told readers what to expect: *The Cloning of a Man*.

In the book Rorvik said that he had been approached by an American millionaire, code-named 'Max', who wished to have himself cloned—in other words, to have a child created from one of his own body cells, so that the child would have exactly the same genetic make-up as he had. Something like this had been done with frogs, but not with mammals. It had never been attempted with humans. Max, however, was prepared to set up a research laboratory to carry out the task. According to Rorvik a willing scientist was found, the attempt was successful, and Max is now a proud father. The infant, instead of being a product of the chance combination of the genetic codes of two individuals, has only one genetic parent. Genetically speaking, Max's son is a carbon copy of his father.

The book provoked an immediate outcry. Of all the new biotechnologies, cloning is the one most likely to send a thrill of horror down our spines. It conjures up images of identical armies of human automata marching remorselessly toward a future in which all individuality is swamped; or else it evokes the spectre of a mad scientist bent on replacing the human race as we know it with a new breed of superhumans designed in accordance with his own distorted standards of superiority.

So it is not surprising that soon after Rorvik's book appeared, three prominent scientists sought an investigation into controls over cloning and related genetic research. A United States Congress subcommittee began hearings on the possibility of human cloning. Other scientists, however, stated flatly that Rorvik must have made it all up. The sceptical view prevailed. A lawsuit led eventually to a US District Court judge describing the book as 'a fraud and a hoax'.

A hoax it may have been, but Rorvik succeeded in arousing public interest in cloning as no straightforward fiction writer could have done. Rorvik was, after all, able to preface his book with a quotation from the Nobel Prize-winning geneticist, Joshua Lederberg, who had said of cloning:

There is nothing to suggest any particular difficulty about accomplishing this in mammals or man, though it will rightly be admired as a technical *tour de force* when it is first accomplished. It places man on the brink of a major evolutionary perturbation.

Is Lederberg right? Even if Rorvik's story was an invention, could what it described be done? And if, or when, it can be done, should it be allowed?

Methods and possibilities

To see how close we are to cloning humans, we have to distinguish two different forms of cloning, one already possible, the other still some time ahead.

Let us go back for a moment to standard *in vitro* fertilization. For the purpose of cloning in its simpler form we are interested in the stage at which the egg has been fertilized in its glass dish and has just gone through its first division. It now consists of two cells. We take this two-cell embryo and, under a microscope, separate the cells (this duplicates the natural process which causes identical twins to be born). We place each cell in conditions suitable for growth. They will continue to grow and each cell will become a child. Like identical twins, these children would share a common genetic constitution. They would be clones.

This form of cloning has already been done with cattle, and healthy identical twin calves produced. There is no technical reason why it could not be done with humans. It works because the cells of an early embryo are not specialized. Later, they will be fixed in different roles: some will become blood cells, some nerve cells, others bone marrow, and so on. For the first few days, however, each cell is totipotent: it has the potential to divide and give rise to all the other cells.

By this method of cloning we can ensure that any child has a genetically identical clone. We cannot, however, make a child that is a genetic carbon-copy of any older person. The clones will be the same age. No mad dictators or eccentric millionaires will therefore be able to clone themselves. The dictator may be all-powerful, but his cells will have lost their totipotency.

There is one qualification to the statement that the clones produced by embryo division will be the same age. If we combine this form of cloning with embryo freezing, the clones could be thawed at different times. They would then vary in age. Suppose a couple had their embryo divided into two clones, had one transferred to the womb, and the other frozen. The transferred embryo would become their first child. Suppose it was a boy. They might wait until he had grown up, and then ask him if he would like to reproduce in the normal way, or would prefer to rear his clone as his own child. If he chose to rear his clone, the other embryo could be thawed and implanted into his wife or any other willing woman. If the child were a girl it would be even more straightforward: she could be made pregnant with her own clone. The result would be no different from being able to clone oneself in the manner allegedly sought by Rorvik's millionaire. The catch is, you can't do this unless your parents have had the foresight to clone you as soon as you were conceived, and to keep your clone or clones on ice until you needed them.

For obvious reasons, this is not the method of cloning Rorvik described, nor is it what the word 'cloning' signifies to popular imagination. For most of us, cloning means taking a cell from a living person—or even from a dead one, as in the popular novel and film *The Boys from Brazil*—and using that cell to produce one or more offspring genetically identical to the person from whom the cell was taken.

Cloning from mature living things is not a new idea. Every time a gardener strikes a cutting, cloning has taken place. (The word 'cloning' comes from a Greek word meaning twig, as one might use for a cutting.) Cuttings are genetically identical to the plants from which they are taken; that is why almost all commercially grown fruit trees are 'clones'—fruit-growers do not want to leave the quality of the fruit to chance.

Cloning from a living animal requires a different technique. To clone a frog, one first takes a frog egg and cuts out the nucleus—the small central element containing the genetic information contributed by the female frog. Then the nucleus of another frog cell is placed into the egg. The egg responds as if it had been fertilized: it grows and develops into a tadpole and ultimately into another frog. This happens because the egg is no longer just an unfertilized egg with only half the genetic information needed to form a complete individual, and therefore requiring a sperm to provide the other half. Instead it now has the full genetic code of the frog cell from which it was taken.

Skilled scientists can carry this out almost routinely, provided the frog cell from which they take the nucleus is an *embryonic* cell. The procedure has been done most often with cells taken from the blastula stage of embryonic growth. At this point the embryo has divided twelve or thirteen times, and consists of thousands of cells. When older embryonic cells are used, the success rate decreases because the cells have become specialized and lost their totipotency. Attempts to use cells from adult frogs have not yet resulted in live frogs; tadpoles have been produced, but all have died.

Using this procedure frogs, toads, and salamanders can all be cloned. These animals are amphibians. They lay relatively large eggs which are fertilized in water and develop naturally outside the body. Applying the same technique to a mammal, whether a mouse or a human, is far more difficult. Mammalian eggs are much smaller and so it is more difficult to take out a nucleus and put another in. In addition, the resulting embryo must be put back inside the mammal.

In 1981 Karl Illmensee of the University of Geneva and an American scientist, Peter Hoppe, claimed the first successful cloning of a mammal. Nuclei taken from a seven-day-old mouse embryo were inserted into mouse eggs from which the nuclei had been removed. The eggs were then implanted into 'surrogate mother' mice, who later gave birth to genetically identical mice. Since this experiment was reported, other scientists have attempted to repeat it, but so far without success.

At the time of writing, therefore, we still find it exceptionally difficult to clone mammals by the transfer of a nucleus from an embryonic cell to an egg whose nucleus has been removed. As for the cloning of a mammal from a cell taken from an adult, this still appears to be some distance ahead, if indeed it will ever prove possible. What would be needed is some means of treating the adult nucleus so that it loses its specialization and regains the ability to create a new individual. Can this be done? So far, the question remains unanswered.

Why clone?

As David Rorvik tells the story in *In His Image*, Max was a man who hated leaving anything to chance. He had never had children by the normal method, because 'the reproductive process, entailing as it did a chance alignment of hereditary factors in a veritable ocean of genes, went against his grain'. Max was proud both of his abilities—he had worked his way to the top—and of his strong physical constitution, which had kept him healthy and vigorous well into what for other men would be old age. He wanted to be sure of passing these qualities on to his child.

The book is a hoax, but its author thought carefully about why someone might want to clone himself, and came up with a plausible reason. There are also other possible motivatons. A sperm bank in California now offers sperm from Nobel Prize-winning scientists and other specially selected high achievers. There have been some takers, women hoping for exceptionally intelligent children. Their hopes may be disappointed, because the children of exeptionally intelligent people are, on average, less intelligent than their parents. This phenomenon, known as 'regression to the mean', is an application of the basic principles of genetics. If an exceptionally intelligent person could be cloned, however, there would be no regression to the mean. In so far as intelligence is controlled by the genes—and the evidence suggests that somewhere between 40 per cent and 80 per cent of variations in IQ are inherited—the clone would have the same intelligence as the person cloned. So if there are women keen to be artificially inseminated by a Nobel Prize-winning sperm donor, presumably there would also be women even more keen to give birth to a clone from such a person.

Cloning would enable single people to have children without making use of genetic material from outsiders. They might dislike the idea of a child who would always carry the genetic legacy of a stranger; and they might think it better for the child not to have an unknown or distant biological parent. To avoid this, a woman could clone herself, as Christine planned to do in our prologue. A man could use a surrogate; there would then be some involvement by another person, but nothing that left a permanent genetic mark on the child. Some infertile couples might wish to clone for the same reason. If the man produces no sperm or the woman no egg, they could have children using AID or donor eggs; but they could avoid the involvement of an outsider by cloning them-selves—to adapt the popular song, a boy from you, a girl from me.

As this last example illustrates, cloning could be used as a method of selecting the sex of one's children. A clone from a man will always be male, and from a woman, always female. There are, however, likely to be simpler methods of sex selection available soon—indeed there are other methods available now. We therefore discuss this issue in a separate section at the end of this chapter.

The test-tube pioneer Robert Edwards has suggested a motivation for the simpler form of cloning, by embryo division at the two-cell stage:

There is [a] compelling reason for dividing embryos in two. One half could be examined to type [to determine the gene type of] the other, especially in families known to be carrying inherited defects. Embryos carrying a defective gene could then be 'aborted *in vitro*' at 5 days of gestation, and a non-defective embryo replaced in the mother. This approach would surely be preferable to the current method of aborting foetuses later in pregnancy.

This technique would require the use of gene probes that could work in minute pieces of tissue: these are already being developed. It is, for instance, already possible to determine the sex of a very early embryo, so this method could already be used for sex selection. The amount of information we can obtain at this early stage is bound to increase steadily in the next few years. As it does, wider possibilities of genetic selection will open up. Edwards envisages using this form of genetic selection 'especially' when a genetic defect is suspected; but if the information were available, it could also be used to select positively for desirable qualities.

A different reason for cloning was mentioned in Chapter 3 of this book. It may prove possible to grow embryos to provide tissues or organs that would save the lives of people dying from a variety of diseases. The major problem with tissue and organ transplants is rejection. This does not occur with donations from identical twins, and it would not occur with a donation from one's own clone. It may turn out that organs taken from embryos at a very early stage, and then grown in culture, are in any case less prone to rejection; or we may learn how to transform the specially cultured tissues so as to suppress the features that cause the tissue to be rejected; but if neither of these prove to be the case, the answer might be to clone embryos from the people who need the new tissue or organ. Alternatively, if cloning from adults remains impracticable, parents may do their children a favour by having them cloned by embryo division at the two-cell stage, and freezing one of the pair. Should the child who results from the other embryo ever need a replacement organ or tissue, there would be a genetically identical embryo in cold storage, ready to be used.

We would guess that at least some of these reasons why people might wish to clone would not arouse much opposition. Those who do not reject abortion altogether will find it difficult to disagree with Edwards's assertion that 'abortion *in vitro*'—in other words, the discarding of a defective embryo before it has been transferred to the womb—is preferable to the birth of a severely defective child, or to an abortion after a test during pregnancy has shown that the child will be defective. Similarly, the provision of tissues or organs that will not be rejected is unquestionably a desirable goal. Nevertheless, some will say that research on cloning should be stopped, because the potential for abuse is too great. These people may fear that once the cloning technique exists, it will become impossible to stop it being used to create identical armies of human automata, all doing the bidding of a totalitarian dictator; or that it will be used to breed a new race of superhumans. So before we take our discussion further, we need to assess the reality of the fears that cloning raises.

Armies of clones?

A cloned person is the same as the individual from which he or she is cloned only in the sense that the book you are now reading is the same as the copy in the library. They are the same book, but different volumes, and different things have happened to them. A clone therefore is not an extension of the individual from which it is cloned, but another, albeit genetically identical, individual. What is true of a single clone is equally true of multiple clones. Such multiples would necessarily have different experiences, and would react to their experiences in their own respective ways. Whether they had similar personalities would depend, as it does with identical twins, on whether their upbringing and environment were more or less similar. Just as 'identical' twins are never really identical in personality, so clones would not be truly identical either.

With this caveat in mind, let us think about the popular image of a cloned army of human automata. Just assuming, for the sake of argument, that somebody did produce a multiple human clone, the people produced would not be automata. They would be separate individuals. Their own brains, not the brain of their progenitor or the scientist who produced them, would control their behaviour, just as surely as our brains control our behaviour.

'But', it might be objected, 'the clones could be programmed by brainwashing.' Well, they might be, but so might anybody. Brainwashing techniques have been known and practised for thousands of years. Modern techniques differ only in their degree of refinement from those practised by religious cults and ruling élites centuries ago. If some mad dictator wished to programme groups of people, it would be a pointless and expensive exercise to have them cloned first. Identical twins are not more susceptible to brainwashing techniques than single births, and no more would cloned individuals be. Those who fear brainwashing techniques creating human automata should not flatter themselves that keeping cloning at bay will limit the risk. Mad dictators will brainwash whoever they get their hands on. To think that they will wait until they can mass-produce groups of physically identical humans is to attribute to them a passion for symmetry which is logically irrelevant to the fulfilment of their evil projects. The solution is to keep power out of the hands of dictators, especially mad ones.

The objector might persist: 'Wouldn't cloned people feel a sense of affinity with one another that the rest of us would not feel? Wouldn't they perhaps even have an ability to communicate with one another that the rest of us lack?' Perhaps they would, but only to the extent that identical twins have, and why would that be bad? The answer will be, of course, that this would bond them together into more efficient armies in the service of a mad dictator. But we return to the point that cloning would be a grossly inefficient way of raising armies. It would take at least eighteen years. Few mad dictators are so patient. Most would prefer to train existing eighteen-year-olds. As for bonding of fighting units, there are other equally effective, and not entirely new, methods of bonding. The Spartans had one way, the Thebans another; Hitler had his way and the Allies theirs. For what it's worth, the relatively less clone-like legions of the Thebans and the World War II Allies were more successful in the long run.

The fear embodied in this particular image of cloning is therefore an over-reaction. The fact that people have the same genetic code ensures that they look alike. But that people look alike does not ensure that they think alike, and it certainly does not make them peculiarly susceptible to brainwashing. Perhaps cloned individuals may have unusual empathy but that does not mean they would lack individuality.

Superclone?

The other popularly invoked image is that of the mad scientist producing a new race of supermen and women. This overlooks the fact that a clone is a copy of, not an improvement on, its original. So cloning cannot produce anything superior to a specimen produced by ordinary sexual reproduction. Of course the fear is that the mad scientist will take one or two superior specimens and reproduce them *en masse*. But superior at what? The world is now so specialized that no single individual could be superior at everything. A nation which cloned its best runner would have to wait about twenty years for its gold medals; and by then a quite different physique might have been found to be superior. At best, the cloned athletes would, for a while, win all the track events their progenitor would have won including, of course, the relay events. They would have their moment, or years, of glory, until one day they would be beaten. For sooner or later the random processes of sexual reproduction would throw up a person with a physical constitution superior in the relevant respects to the person from whom the clones were taken.

The situation would be similar if a nation decided to clone its best scientist or thinker. Once the cloning was done, there would still be many a slip twixt the cup and the lip. We can assume that the genetic code constitutes at least some part of the ingredients of genius, so that the cloned intellectuals would have a good prospect of achieving academic distinction. In order to reproduce an intelligence like that of Einstein or Bertrand Russell, however, a nation would need to reproduce the cultural and educational environment which enabled their genius to flourish in the first place. Given the passage of time and the uniqueness of individual circumstances, this might prove impossible. In any case, the random mutations of the gene pool, and the rough and tumble of intellectual life, would sooner or later throw up a greater genius than the clones.

Mass production of clones would be unwise. Cloning does not allow for genetic improvement. It cannot do so, because its principle is replication, not change. Clones could of course be trained for feats for which their original had no aptitude, and they might well be suitable material for such training; but the random processes of sexual reproduction will sooner or later produce even more suitable material. That is why cloning cannot replace the natural diversity of the human gene pool. Once the gene pool has produced a superior specimen, limited cloning could perhaps usefully multiply ten- or twenty-fold the resources which an accident of nature had conferred on one individual. But a nation which relied only on cloning for the production of superior individuals would eventually dwindle to second rank, because elsewhere even more superior specimens will be produced in the unpredictable way they have been produced since time began. Where evolution is concerned, there is no substitute for hetero-sexual reproduction.

So far we have been at pains to emphasize that cloned people would still be individuals. Members of a multiple clone would be physically as alike as identical twins, while similarity in personality would be affected by whether their upbringing and environment were similar. A world in which there were a mass production of clones would therefore be like a world in which women started giving birth, in large numbers of batches, to quintuplets, sextuplets, or whatever, with the siblings being split up and adopted out into different families. Now the question is, would such a world be better or worse than the one we now live in? The answer will partly depend on what these multiple births have to contribute to civilization. But this contribution has to be weighed against the fact that cloned individuals, to the extent that they are similar in personality, talent, disposition, and so on, will reduce the pool of diversity available to any society. A few multiple clones here and there would reduce this diversity only to an insignificant degree, and this insignificant loss likewise would have to be weighed against the contributions they might make. But a substantial inroad into the diversity of a society would have quite undesirable consequences.

When, for example, a problem is to be solved it is frequently the case that no one individual has a monopoly on all the good ideas. In fact the reverse is sometimes true: people of radically different viewpoints each have something of value to contribute, and these contributions are possible precisely because of the radical diversity of their points of view. There is also a connection between this fruitful diversity and yet another diversity—differences in ways of living. The fact that A lives her life in a different way from B shows B that his way is not the only way. Such experiments in living, as John Stuart Mill called them, provoke thought, and are part of the generative pool of diversity which has served the human race well in the past.

To whatever extent cloning reduced this diversity, to that extent it would reduce the viability of humanity. If there were multiple clones, to whatever extent they thought alike and viewed the world in the same way, to that extent they would be denied (and would be denying everyone else) the benefits of diversity. If the human species, or any other species, were one big clone, a single infection could wipe out the whole race. If every suggestion box in every work-place contained only the same endlessly repeated suggestion, the human race might not survive a crisis in which off-beat ideas were needed. It would certainly not progress as fast as it would if the suggestions were more varied.

So fears of cloning are based on far-fetched scenarios. These fears do not justify a ban on all further research into cloning. On the other hand, cloning does involve reducing the number of baskets into which we are putting our eggs. We should not put *too* many eggs in the one basket. If cloning were to become a reality, it would have to be kept within strict limits.

The cloned individual

Although thinking about cloning does not give us nightmares, it raises other problems which, we think, would make it inadvisable in most cases. The major objection to cloning genuises would be one that also holds against its closest existing analogue, artificial insemination by Nobel Prize-winning donor. It is the psychological pressure that could be experienced by a child who fails to live up to expectations. In the case of the sperm bank we mentioned earlier, this failure to accomplish as much as one's father is likely to happen as a result of the genetic lottery. Cloning rules out that cause, but does not rule out environmental factors which could be responsible for a cloned child not having the abilities of the person from whom the genetic information was taken. Parents might do all they can to ensure that the cloned child has every educational advantage, but they could not possibly know what the particular genetic constitution of their child needed to reach its peak—it might even need to battle against tremendous adversity!

Parents who had gone to considerable trouble to obtain a clone of a brilliant scientist or leading statesman would not find it easy to hide their disappointment in a child who lacked the qualities they thought to guarantee. Would they be able to love their children with the uncritical love of parents who accept their children for what they are—a love which does not depend on the extent to which the children measure up to some preconceived standard of excellence? And will the children not suffer from the knowledge that they are not living up to their parents' expectations? Of course, many children know that they are not living up to their parents' expectations; but the impact would be immeasurably greater if the child knew that its parents had gone to the trouble of ensuring that it had all the genetic characteristics necessary for the expected, but unattained, level of achievement.

We wonder, too, about other personal relationships of cloned individuals. If a particular person had been cloned many times, so that there were several genetically identical copies in the community, would this lead to oddities in their friendships and their love lives? In a 1982 BBC Television programme entitled *Brave New Babies*, the Oxford philosopher Jonathan Glover raised this question. To investigate it he found the nearest thing to a set of cloned people: a set of identical triplets. The triplets, male and around eighteen years old, all had girlfriends. Glover asked the girls whether they felt equally attracted to all three of the boys. The girls said they did not. (One of them admitted to hugging the wrong triplet, but only in error.) Glover then asked if it would make a difference if instead of their boyfriends having two identical brothers, they had forty. The girls blanched: not surprisingly, they were unsure of the answer.

These doubts about cloning may be misplaced. Parents may soon adjust their expectations and love their cloned children for what they are, just as parents who hope for a child of one sex come to dote on the child that turns out to be of the other sex. Other relationships may prove no more difficult for forty identical clones than for three identical triplets. Nevertheless, these doubts should be given some weight.

Should cloning be banned?

The Australian National Health and Medical Research Council guide-lines which accept IVF, egg donation, and embryo freezing, appear to draw the line at cloning:

Cloning experiments designed to produce from human tissues viable or potentially viable offspring that are multiple and genetically identical are ethically unacceptable.

The parallel British body, the British Medical Research Council, did not mention cloning at all in its research guide-lines; but the British Medical Association's statement of May 1983 takes a similar line to the Australian guide-lines:

It is not ethically acceptable for medical practitioners to be involved in *in vitro* fertilisation and embryo replacement procedures in which the gametes (sperm or ova), embryos, or parts thereof are subjected to manipulations, including procedures designed to change their genetic make up or to induce the formation of multiple progeny ('cloning'), if there is any intent to transfer the resulting embryos to a uterus.

These statements have been widely interpreted—both in the popular press and in more specialized journals—as ruling out human cloning. For instance, the *Hastings Center Report*, perhaps the world's leading bioethics periodical, reported simply that the Australian guide-lines 'consider cloning . . . as "ethically unacceptable" '. Anyone who has followed our previous discussion, however, will have no difficulty in seeing that the passages just quoted are more remarkable for what they do not prohibit than for what they do. Both statements reject the formation of *multiple* cloned individuals. The British statement, in its general reference to the genetic manipulation of sperm, eggs, or embryos, would also rule out the production of a single cloned individual. The Australian guide-lines say nothing against cloning that is not intended to produce multiple offspring, and so would not exclude research designed to enable someone like David Rorvik's 'Max' to have one cloned child.

More significant still, at least for the immediate future, is the fact that neither statement seeks to stop cloning by embryo division to allow gene typing. Nor is there any prohibition of cloning to provide spare parts. The British statement is compatible with both these procedures because neither would involve the transfer of the resulting embryo to the uterus. The Australian guide-lines do not stand in the way, because even though the embryos might be regarded as 'potentially viable offspring', they do not—or at least they need not—involve the production of *multiple* genetically identical embryos.

We agree that in discussing whether cloning experiments should continue, it is important to distinguish between work that is aimed at producing living human beings and work that has no such intention. The most powerful reasons for cloning are to enable embryos to be genetically typed, and to provide compatible tissues and organs for medical purposes. Moreover, the objections to cloning are weakest when directed against these forms of cloning. Since neither leads to a living human being, we can disregard objections based on the risk of an abnormal child, or on the psychological problems that might face a cloned person. The major remaining ethical objection is that the rights of the embryo would not be respected; but we dealt with this objection in Chapter 3. For the reasons given there, we do not share the concern expressed by the Australian guide-lines over the production of 'potentially viable offspring'. We would rather see the line drawn at sentience than at potential viability, which could be interpreted as applying to the very earliest embryos.

Cloning designed to allow gene typing and the subsequent selection of embryos must also face the objections that have been brought against other forms of genetic engineering—that it is 'playing God', or interfering with evolution, or that it will be impossible to find the correct criteria for selection. Since we consider genetic engineering in the next chapter, we shall postpone discussion of these issues. Meanwhile we can provisionally conclude that, the genetic engineering issues apart, this form of cloning should be permitted.

The use of embryos for spare parts was discussed in Chapter 3 and found acceptable within the limits there specified. We have now seen that the idea of cloning these embryos raises no significant new objection, and therefore it too can be accepted.

What of the distinction between single and multiple cloning? The Australian guide-lines appear to give it considerable weight: the British do not. Should millionaires like Max be permitted to make one genetic copy of themselves, but not two? Or should they not be permitted to make any at all? And should single people or infertile couples be allowed to use cloning to avoid the use of donor sperm or eggs? Again, the Australian guide-lines appear to permit it, as long as no more than one child is cloned from each adult: the British guide-lines say that it is not ethically acceptable.

The grounds for producing cloned individuals are much less convincing than the case for cloning to allow gene typing or to provide spare parts. The desires of single people or infertile couples to have children are weighty enough, but they can be satisfied without resorting to cloning. The desire to avoid the use of donor sperm or eggs seems much less fundamental, and we would expect its frustration to produce correspondingly less misery. We are even less impressed with the desires of someone like Max, who wants to produce a genetic replica of himself rather than leave anything to chance.

Would these forms of cloning be more acceptable if there were some guarantee that only one clone of each adult would be produced? This would eliminate the—in any case unlikely—prospect of an army of clones. It would also allay fears that cloning will lead to eerie crowds of innumerable identical people. Of greater ethical significance, perhaps, is the fact that it would avoid the psychological and personal problems that might face members of large identical sets of cloned people. Other psychological problems, however, would remain a serious enough risk to outweigh the desires some people may have for a child that is 'their own' in a way no child has ever been up to now.

Some will argue that even though a government might consider these reasons for cloning inadequate, and might therefore properly refuse to assist in any way, it is quite another matter for the government to prohibit these forms of cloning. This latter step, we can imagine Max saying, would be an unjustified interference with the private decisions of individuals who are not violating anyone's rights. Hence the State should leave people free to clone themselves if they wish to do so, and can afford to pay for it themselves.

The first retort to come to mind is that Max's plan did affect one other non-consenting party: his cloned offspring. The problem with this retort is that it might justify too much. Any decision to reproduce affects the child that will result, and that child cannot consent to the decision. In our anxiety to prevent Max from cloning himself, are we using an argument which could lead to the State having the right to license all reproduction?

We believe that the State can be justified in interfering with decisions to reproduce, either in order to control population growth or to prevent practices which might disadvantage the children born. But we also believe that the State should interfere only in the most extreme cases. For instance, the State would be justified in preventing the genetic manipulation of embryos designed to produce the equivalent of the Epsilons of *Brave New World*. Cloning does not appear to be so extreme a case. Max can plausibly argue that his son will receive the benefit of a genetically sound constitution, predisposed to robust health and an above average intelligence. True, the child may have some difficulty in adjusting to his special circumstances; but on balance his prospects for a happy and fulfilling life are at least as good as those of children born in more ordinary circumstances.

We find this claim difficult to deny. It assumes, of course, that the cloned individual will turn out as planned, without gross defects. The risk of something going drastically wrong is, at present, a sufficient reason for the State to prevent individuals from cloning themselves. Should it one day be shown that this can be done without risk, we would reluctantly concede that while the government should not assist in the process, perhaps it should not prohibit it either, as long as it is limited to one replica per person.

The remaining justification for producing cloned individuals is based not on the desires of individuals who wish to clone themselves, but on the advantages to all of us that would come from multiplying the number of people possessing rare and valuable abilities. This points toward multiple, rather than single, cloning, for if each person with special abilities were cloned once only, the expected benefits would be considerably reduced. The production of 'limited editions' of twenty or even fifty or a hundred clones of exceptionally gifted people, widely distributed throughout the nation, would maximize the gains without significantly reducing the vital diversity of the gene pool.

Since this form of cloning involves the production of multiple clones, it falls outside both the Australian and the British guidelines. This is not surprising, for in addition to the concern about cloning itself, it raises the very sensitive issue of attempting to improve the genetic constitution of the human species. Only if it were agreed that this attempt is desirable would it be appropriate to consider whether cloning is the right way to go about it. As we discuss this issue in the following chapter, we shall put off, until then, any further consideration of this sort of cloning. Meanwhile we turn to an issue raised indirectly by cloning, but also of independent interest.

Boy or girl: should we choose?

Since ancient times we have tried to choose the sex of our children. Aristotle advised those wanting a boy to wait until the wind is in the north before having intercourse. Every folk culture has its own techniques, from sex with boots on to hanging one's trousers on the left side of the bed for a girl, and the right side for a boy. Recently some supposedly more scientific methods have been suggested. Landrum Shettles, the controversial New York gynaecologist whose attempt to produce the world's first IVF baby was frustrated by his hospital chief (see p. 47) has claimed that by correct timing of intercourse and the use of vaginal douches, (acidic for girls, alkaline for boys) any couple can give themselves an 80 per cent chance of getting a child of the sex they desire. Shettles has co-authored a book, *Choose Your Baby's Sex*, setting out his method. The other co-author is David Rorvik.

If we succeeded in cloning adults, one side-effect would be a 100 per cent reliable way of selecting the sex of one's child. A cloned child would always be the same sex as the person from which it was cloned. Of course, it would also be the same in so many other respects that for many parents this method would be a severe case of overkill. Technically, too, cloning adults to select sex is a bit like using a laser beam to open letters. Simpler methods are either already feasible, or soon will be.

One way of selecting sex presents no technical difficulties at all. When a pregnant woman has a higher than normal risk of bearing a defective child—for example, if she is over thirty-five—it is now standard practice to check the foetus by a procedure known as amniocentesis. This involves drawing off a small amount of the amniotic fluid surrounding the foetus. The amniotic fluid will contain cells from the foetus, and these can be examined for abnormalities. The examination also reveals the sex of the foetus. If a serious defect is revealed, the woman will be offered an abortion. If no abnormalities are detected, the doctor will often ask the woman if she wishes to know whether her child is a boy or a girl. Many prefer to wait until the baby is born, and those who do wish to know are generally motivated by nothing more significant than the desire to begin knitting bootees of the right colour. There have been cases, however, of couples who have sought amniocentesis precisely in order to find out the sex of the foetus, with a view to aborting it if it is not the sex they want.

Many doctors will not perform amniocentesis if they believe it is being requested with a view to sex selection; but how can one prevent deception? A couple may claim that one partner has a family history of haemophilia, and so they do not want to risk a male child (only males suffer from haemophilia). If a male child is in fact what they want, then after the amniocentesis report assures them that the child is female, they can go elsewhere for an abortion. It seems, however, that such behaviour is rare. One American genetics centre announced that it was prepared to perform amniocentesis for sex selection if, after counselling, the client requested it. Six months later the centre had received only one request. The lesson appears to be that while many couples would like to select the sex of their offspring, very few are so determined to do so that they are prepared to abort a healthy foetus of the 'wrong' sex.

Couples might be more inclined to reject an embryo of the unwanted sex if it could be done without abortion. Cloning by dividing the early embryo would make this possible, for we can already determine the sex of the newly fertilized embryo. One embryo of each divided pair could be used to reveal the sex of the other member of the pair, which could then be transferred to the womb or discarded, as the couple wished. The woman is spared an abortion; on the other hand she has to submit to all the complications of IVF. Unless IVF becomes easier, less expensive, and more reliable, this method would not be attractive to couples who can conceive in the normal way.

This method of embryo sex selection might be of more interest to infertile couples, who in any case need IVF if they are to have children. Of those responding to our questionnaire, however, only about a quarter said that they would like the scientists to be able to select the sex of the embryo before transfer. Nearly all the remainder—72 per cent—did not want this done. Scientists at several different centres around the world are close to finding a simpler method, applicable for all couples. The sex of the child is determined by the sperm that fertilizes the egg. Sperm carrying an X chromosome produce girls, and sperm carrying a Y chromosome produce boys. The female-producing sperm are larger than the male-producing sperm, and also give out slightly different electrical charges. From time to time, scientists announce promising results in separating the sperm. The methods of separation include spinning in a centrifuge, using a weak electrical current to attract sperm of one electrical charge, and suspending the sperm in a fluid in the hope that the female-producing sperm will settle nearer the bottom. In May 1983 Professor Hiroshi Nakajima of the Tokyo Medical and Dental University claimed the best results so far: using electrical separation, he had produced 100 per cent pure X-sperm and 83 per cent pure Y-sperm. If these results are confirmed, sex selection by means of sperm separation and artificial insemination would not be far ahead; and since artificial insemination is easy and painless, this method would be much more likely to be widely used than methods requiring either abortion or IVF.

Should sex selection be allowed? The major objection is that it would lead to an imbalance of the sexes, most likely a preponderance of males. This would, of course, vary from society to society. Some cultures have taken their preference for boys to such lengths that unwanted female babies were killed at birth. Others are indifferent between the two sexes. Surveys of American families indicate a slight preference for boys. Amitai Etzioni, professor of sociology at Columbia University, estimates that if reliable sex selection methods were available in America, at least 54.75 children in every hundred born would be males. This means a surplus of males over females of 9.5 per cent. The imbalance would probably be much greater in countries which place a higher value on having a son. On the other hand once the shortage of females became apparent the value placed on daughters might rise.

The only evidence about the effects of an uneven sex ratio comes from societies affected by special factors. Throughout the early period of white settlement, Australia had substantially more males than females: the same is true of the American West, and of Israel in the early immigration periods. Conversely, after World War II both the USSR and Germany had many more females than males. One might tentatively conclude that more males means a higher crime rate and good business for prostitutes; but it is virtually impossible to generalize across diverse historical and cultural circumstances.

Is the satisfaction of the desire of parents for children of a particular sex worth the cost? Etzioni points out that even if we are not alarmist about the overall social consequences, we have to consider the surplus males—some 360,000 born every year in the United States, if Etzioni's figures are right—who, unable to find a mate, would have to make do with prostitution, homosexuality, enforced celibacy, or polyandry. The joys experienced by parents who would have children of the sex they wanted would, Etzioni believes, be much less intensely felt than the sorrows of the males who could not find mates.

Landrum Shettles has denied that sex selection will lead to any long-term imbalance of the sexes. He thinks most couples want evenly balanced families, and an abundance of one sex would soon lead to the other sex becoming more popular. Moreover, Shettles sees positive advantages in sex selection as a means of controlling population growth. In this he is supported by Paul Ehrlich, author of *The Population Bomb*, who has urged the setting up of a Bureau of Population and Environment which would, among other things, encourage research into sex determination. As Ehrlich puts it:

. . . if a simple method could be found to guarantee that first-born children were males, then population control measures in many areas would be somewhat eased. In our country and elsewhere, couples with only female children 'keep trying' in hope of a son.

No doubt some families with only male children also 'keep trying'! Sex selection would have an especially pronounced effect in countries like India, where many couples try to have at least two sons; sex selection would halve the number of children the average couple need to produce in order to have two sons. In China, too, the 'one-child' policy has been threatened by the traditional belief that only a male child can carry on the family line. Many families refused to stop at one child if the first child proved to be a girl. When officials took punitive measures in order to enforce the policy, reports started coming in of female infanticide. Since the population explosion is arguably the greatest problem facing the world today, any method that offers a hope of containing it should not be rejected except on the clearest and most serious grounds.

One way of obtaining the gains offered by sex selection without suffering the disadvantages would be for the use of the method to be monitored, and steps taken to prevent any significant imbalance. If the method of sex selection were available only through registered medical practitioners, control could be kept by setting up waiting-lists for those who wanted a child of the sex that was being chosen too frequently. Couples who were more interested in having a child soon than in having one of the right sex would drop off the waiting-list, and an even sex ratio would be restored without frustrating the desires of those prepared to wait.

It would be less easy to control a 'do-it-yourself' method like that recommended by Shettles. This is not a problem with Shettles's method itself, since the measures required are irksome and its efficacy is doubtful. It could become a problem, however, if some future technique should prove both simple and reliable. Then the government would have to try publicizing the developing imbalance and warning parents of the risk that a child of the sex in demand would be unable to find a mate. If this did not work, as a last resort couples might have to be taxed in accordance with the number of children they have of the preponderant sex.

Monitoring the sex ratio and warning of imbalances might be enough to avoid most of the problems of a grossly uneven ratio of males to females. In any case, the seriousness of these problems is difficult to estimate; whereas the seriousness of continued population growth is undeniable. Countries facing famine as a result of over-population might choose unfettered selection as a means of stopping population growth. In this way the good achieved by a convenient method of sex selection is likely to be more significant than any harm it would cause.

7 GENETIC ENGINEERING

Some thirty-five years ago physicists learned how to manipulate the forces in the nucleus of the atom, and the world has been struggling to cope with the results of that discovery ever since. The ability to penetrate the nucleus of the living cell, to rearrange and transplant the nucleic acids that constitute the genetic material of all forms of life, seems a more beneficient power but one that is likely to prove at least as profound in its consequences.

Nicholas Wade, *The Ultimate Experiment*

In this chapter we look at one last topic related to the development of IVF. It is the most far-reaching of all, for it opens up the prospect of reshaping the human species.

Genetic engineering is a loose term. Some use it to mean any kind of deliberate tinkering with the human gene pool. So defined, it includes eugenics schemes which go back as far as Plato, whose ideal republic would have encouraged 'union between the better specimens of both sexes' while limiting the reproduction of the less desirable types. This form of genetic engineering needs no new technology at all. At the other end of the spectrum there are the latest techniques of manufacturing recombinant DNA and splicing genes to produce entirely new forms of life. We shall describe these techniques later in this chapter.

In between these extremes lie various methods of genetic selection using modern techniques that are less far-reaching than gene splicing. For instance, pre-natal diagnosis is now being widely used to detect genetic abnormalities during pregnancy. An abortion is performed if the test shows an abnormal foetus. This will have an effect on the genetic inheritance of future generations; but the main effect will be to restore the process of natural selection that used to operate before modern medicine found the means to save the lives of many genetically abnormal children.

The next step may be the use of IVF combined with cloning by cell division at the two-cell stage, as described in the previous chapter, so that one embryo of a genetically identical pair can be examined. An embryo discovered to be defective would be rejected, a normal embryo would be transferred to the womb. With artificial stimulation to produce several embryos, this procedure could easily be taken a step further. Each embryo would be divided, and one of each pair examined. As our ability to 'read' the genetic constitution of the embryo improves, the basis on which parents would be able to select the embryo they would most like to develop into their child will increase. Ultimately this method could be used not just to avoid genetic defects, but to select the positive genetic characteristics wanted by the parents.

In keeping with the theme of this book, the present chapter will focus on methods of genetic engineering made possible or foreseeable by recent developments in biology and medicine. Hence we shall be more concerned with new methods of manipulating genes than with old-fashioned eugenics—although some of the old issues re-emerge with the new technology.

The ability to manipulate genes is not itself a consequence of IVF or any other developments in human reproduction. Splicing bacteria to create new life forms that will devour oil spills; engineering plants that can surpass all existing cereals in the efficiency with which they convert sunlight to nourishment for humans; producing cattle that grow rapidly to twice the normal size—that these things are coming closer has no direct connection with IVF. What IVF has done, however, is to open the way to applying these techniques to human beings; and that, for many people, is the most frightening prospect of all.

Creating new forms of life has traditionally been the prerogative of gods. The dream of discovering this secret is an old one—but so is the thought that this dream could turn into a nightmare. In sixteenth-century Prague, the renowned Rabbi Loew was said to have taken a handful of dust and created a gigantic monster called a Golem, which roamed the streets bringing vengeance to those who persecuted the Jews. Early in the nineteenth century Mary Wollstonecraft Shelley captured the public imagination with a novel which told the tragic tale of Victor Frankenstein, a young scientist who discovered how to create life, but unwittingly made a half-human monster. The monster killed all Frankenstein's nearest and dearest and finally drove him to his death in a state of half-mad despair. The moral of the story is made explicit by Frankenstein's response to the ship's captain who serves as narrator of the novel. Frankenstein, now near death, has given the captain a full account of his life, except for one crucial detail:

Sometimes I endeavoured to gain from Frankenstein the particulars of his creature's formation: but on this point he was impenetrable. 'Are you mad, my friend?' said he; 'or whither does your senseless curiosity lead you? Would you also create for yourself and the world a demoniacal enemy? Peace, peace! learn my miseries, and do not seek to increase your own.'

Leading scientists now echo the words written by Mary Shelley. Erwin Chargaff, a biologist who did pioneering work in the understanding of DNA, has, like Frankenstein, been critical of following 'curiosity' wherever it may take us:

Have we the right to counteract, irreversibly, the evolutionary wisdom of millions of years, in order to satisfy the curiosity of a few scientists? The future will curse us for it.

Robert Sinsheimer, Chairman of the Department of Biology at the California Institute of Technology, and once an advocate of genetic engineering, also seems to share Victor Frankenstein's view when he asks:

Do we want to assume the basic responsibility for life on this planet—to develop new living forms for our own purposes? Shall we take into our hands our own future evolution? . . . Perverse as it may, initially, seem to the scientist, we must face the fact that there can be unwanted knowledge.

In keeping with the lesson of *Frankenstein*, most people have grave reservations about scientists dabbling with new forms of life. A survey carried out in 1980 by the United States National Science Foundation showed that while most Americans did not think there should be restrictions on scientific research, 'a notable exception was the opposition to scientists creating new life forms'. Almost two-thirds of those questioned thought that studies in this area should not be pursued.

Yet there is a different point of view. If the creation of new forms of life seems a god-like power, what more noble goal can humanity have than to aspire to it? Like Prometheus, the mythical Greek hero who defied the gods and stole from them the secret of fire, should we not challenge the gods and make their powers our own? Or to put it in more scientific terms, should we allow ourselves to remain at the mercy of genetic accident and blind evolution, when we have before us the prospect of acquiring supremacy over the very forces that have created us? Mary Shelley was clearly aware of these god-defying ambitions, for the full title of her novel is *Frankenstein, or the Modern Prometheus*; but if she thus intended to warn us against Promethean ambitions, may she not have been overly pessimistic? Against her imaginative novel we can place the sober report of a United States body with the impressive title of 'President's Commission for the Study of Ethical Problems in Medicine and Biomedical and Behavioral Research'. According to the Commission's report on genetic engineering, 'as a product of human investigation and ingenuity, the new knowledge is a celebration of human creativity, and the new powers are a reminder of human obligations to act responsibly'.

What it is and how it works

How did we come into possesson of the knowledge that poses such an awesome choice?

To begin at the beginning, in genetics, we do not have to go back very far. The laws of inheritance are generally attributed to Gregor Mendel, a nineteenth-century Moravian monk who studied peas in his monastery garden; but Mendel knew nothing about the mechanism which produced the patterns of inheritance he observed. Moreover, the importance of his work went unrecognized until the present century.

Coincidentally, deoxyribonucleic acid, better known as DNA, was discovered around the same time. Johann Miescher, a young Swiss scientist studying in Germany, was exploring the chemistry of the nuclei of living cells. He reported finding an acidic compound consisting of very large molecules. But he had no idea of its function or importance. (At the risk of arousing superstitious fears, we report a more ominous coincidence: fifty years earlier,

Mary Shelley had given Victor Frankenstein's place of birth as Switzerland, and sent him off to study in Germany, where he made his discovery.)

It was not until the 1920s and 30s that evidence began to accumulate proving that DNA somehow passed on inherited characteristics from one generation to the next. *How* this happened remained a mystery until 1953, when, in a celebrated piece of scientific detective work, James Watson and Francis Crick suggested that DNA consisted of a 'double helix'. A helix is simply a spiral, and the structure of DNA is that of two spirals, matching each other like the two sides of a zip.

To understand how this structure explains inheritance, we need to know that although every living cell contains DNA, the precise nature of the DNA varies from one life form to another. It varies in the sequence of four substances within the DNA molecule. These four substances are known by the letters A, G, C, and T, and they can be thought of as the alphabet in which genetic information is written. The precise form of DNA in any one living being can replicate itself, because each strand of the double helix can act as a chemical template or pattern from which a matching second strand can be formed. It is as if the zip were to unzip and each side to produce a model of the other side with which it could unite and form a complete zip identical to the original one. Or as Francis Crick explained it:

The two chains of the DNA, which fit together as a hand fits into a glove, are separated in some way and the hand then acts as a mould for the formation of a new glove while the glove acts as a mould for a new hand. Thus we finish up with two gloved hands where we had only one before.

The next step was to crack the genetic code by which DNA passes on its information and forms the proteins that control the chemical reactions which sustain all living beings. Different proteins consist of different amino acids, and DNA works by specifying the order of amino acids, thus causing specific proteins to be created. There is an intermediary, consisting of another acid, 'messenger ribonucleic acid' or mRNA. The four varying substances in DNA—A, G, C, and T—are transformed in mRNA into combinations of three: we might say that the genetic language is written in words consisting of three letters, drawn from an alphabet of only four letters. This provides sixty-four possible combinations, more than enough to specify the twenty amino acids which, in an enormous variety of combinations and sequences, constitute all the proteins made by living cells.

Once Watson and Crick had explained the structure of DNA, the cracking of the genetic code took another thirteen years work. By 1966 the job was done. The deciphered code confirmed the unity and common origin of all living things, for it turned out to be identical in cabbages and in kings, not to mention viruses and other nasties. This was, in truth, the secret of all life.

A scientific mystery had been solved, but it took a few more years for techniques to be found that could make use of the new knowledge. 'Gene splicing', as it has now developed, uses naturally occurring enzymes which have the ability to break or cut a double strand of DNA. The cut occurs in such a manner that one of the two intertwined strands overlaps the other: this is referred to as a 'sticky end', because it will join up with a separate double strand that has been cut by the same enzyme and has a matching overlap. When two different pieces of DNA are cut and combined in this manner, we have what is called 'recombinant DNA', a new piece of genetic information which, when correctly inserted into a living organism, has the capacity to reproduce itself and pass on its genetic message to its descendents.

The first application of gene splicing was to produce medical products such as insulin and interferon. Up to now insulin for diabetics has been collected from the pancreas glands of cows and pigs. Now it is possible to splice the gene for producing human insulin into a bacterium, which will then produce human insulin. Since bacteria multiply very rapidly, large quantities of insulin can be harvested. In 1982, insulin produced in this manner was approved for sale in the United States and Britain, although technical difficulties still limit its availability.

Interesting and important as this work may be, it has no direct connection with IVF or human reproduction. It is the bacteria which do the reproducing. But gene splicing techniques can be used directly on humans in two different ways: one highly relevant to our topic, and the other not.

The form of gene therapy that is not relevant to human reproduction attempts to treat genetically defective cells in patients suffering from a disease. For instance, sickle-cell anaemia is the result of a defective haemoglobin gene which expresses itself in malfunctioning bone marrow cells. In theory these genetically defective cells could be removed, treated with DNA that would instruct the cells to function normally, and then returned to the patient. This, if it worked—so far it has not—would cure the patient's disease. It would not, however, affect the genetic information such patients carried in every other cell of their bodies. Only the bone marrow cells would have been changed. The germ cells—the sperm or eggs—would still pass on the disease to the patients' descendants, under the normal laws of inheritance.

Suppose, however, that normal haemoglobin gene DNA could be inserted into otherwise defective embryos at a very early stage, before the cells had differentiated themselves according to their various functions. Then all the cells of the resulting individuals would be entirely normal. They would not suffer from the disease, nor would they pass it on to their descendants. The disease might, eventually, be wiped out.

In vitro fertilization makes this a possibility. It means that the embryo is exposed, available for genetic manipulation, at the crucial stage when it is normally inaccessible in the womb. So once normal haemoglobin gene DNA can be isolated and multiplied by the usual gene splicing techniques, it could be injected into the fertilized egg, which would then be transferred to the womb in the normal manner.

Simple as this sounds, it has its problems. Most importantly, normal haemoglobin gene DNA cannot be put into the correct place in the overall genetic code of the embryo. There is no known technique for achieving such precision, and since the total amount of genetic information carried by humans amounts to around 5,000 million DNA 'letters', it seems unlikely that such a technique will be found in the near future. All that can be done is to use the 'shotgun' method: insert the DNA into the nucleus of the cell—even this requires microsurgical techniques—and hope that some will be taken up at the right place, and it will be rejected everywhere else. This is not an idle hope, for some animal experiments have given encouraging results; but they have also made it clear that things do not always go entirely to plan. In one experiment, for instance, rat genes for growth hormone were injected into mouse eggs. The resulting mice were much larger than normal—although the extra growth hormone turned out to be produced from the liver rather than the pituitary gland as it normally would be.

The risk of doing such work on humans would be great. Nor does it seem necessary. If two carriers of a recessive gene, like the sickle-cell gene, have a child, there is only one chance in four that their child will suffer from the disease (two out of four, on average, will be carriers like their parents, while the fourth will be completely normal). Since these inherited conditions can now be detected early in pregnancy, it seems simpler and less risky to use pre-natal diagnosis coupled with abortion, if the diagnosis is positive. Of course, those opposed to abortion will not agree; but they are also unlikely to agree to something as experimental as genetic manipulation of the embryo.

As we have seen, the development of IVF offers a further possibility, again without the risk of genetic manipulation: carriers of genetic diseases could use IVF, with artificial stimulation so that several embryos are produced. These could then be genetically screened, and only those without defect transferred to the mother. For the foreseeable future, this appears a much more realistic means of eliminating defects in humans than does the use of gene splicing techniques.

The ethical issues

We now turn to the ethical issues raised by modern genetic engineering techniques. What we say will, unless the context rules it out, apply not only to gene splicing, but also to embryo typing and selection, or any other method that can achieve the same results.

The safety debate

The first expressions of alarm about research on recombinant DNA had nothing to do with the use of the technique in humans, or indeed with any deliberate application of it. The fear was that bacteria genetically modified for experimental purposes might escape from the laboratory and wreak havoc among living creatures who would have no resistance to it. The danger seemed real enough in 1974 for scientists to accept a self-imposed moratorium on work on recombinant DNA. The United States Government then set up a Recombinant DNA Advisory Committee, which allowed research to go ahead under strict guidelines.

The Committee is still in existence, although the guide-lines have been relaxed. The general consensus of current scientific opinion is that the original fears were exaggerated. 'Crippled' strains of bacteria are now being used, designed to be unable to survive outside the special environment of the laboratory. Careful checks of laboratory workers have failed to reveal infection by the new organisms. No doubt there is still a need for caution, and for continued monitoring of this type of research; but opposition to it continuing at all appears to have ceased.

Quite separate from the issue of the safety of research into recombinant DNA, are questions about the desirability of such research, assuming that it can be carried out safely. Here we reach some ethical objections more akin to those considered in earlier chapters of this book.

Playing God

When the President's Commission for the Study of Ethical Problems in Medicine and Biomedical and Behavioral Research began to examine genetic engineering, it did so at the request of three religious leaders—the General Secretaries of the National Council of Churches, the Synagogue Council of America, and the United States Catholic Conference. In a joint letter, the three General Secretaries warned that once genetic engineering was technically possible, 'Those who would play God will be tempted as never before.'

The President's Commission asked the three religious leaders to elaborate on any specifically religious objections to gene splicing in humans. They in turn appointed theologians to address the Commission. The outcome, as reported by the Commission, was hardly what one would have expected from the General Secretaries' warnings about 'playing God':

In the view of the theologians, contemporary developments in molecular biology raise issues of responsibility rather than being matters to be prohibited because they usurp powers that human beings should not possess. The Biblical religions teach that human beings are, in some sense, co-creators with the Supreme Creator. Thus, as interpreted for the Commission by their representatives, these major religious faiths respect and encourage the enhancement of knowledge about nature, as well as responsible use of that knowledge. Endorsement of genetic engineering, which is praised for its potential to improve the human estate, is linked with the recognition that the misuse of human freedom creates evil and human knowledge and power can result in harm.

So even from a religious point of view, genetic engineering is not to be rejected outright. It may be used 'to improve the human estate'.

Rejecting the wisdom of evolution

We saw earlier that Erwin Chargaff and Robert Sinsheimer—both scientists doing research with DNA—warned against meddling with evolution. Chargaff suggested that 'the future will curse us' if we irreversibly counteract 'the evolutionary wisdom of millions of years in order to satisfy the curiosity of a few scientists'. Is this perhaps a more compelling, secular revision of the injunction against playing God? Putting aside the obviously false claim that genetic engineering serves only to satisfy curiosity, is there any truth in the assertion that to engage in genetic engineering is to risk upsetting the evolutionary applecart?

Humans have been interfering with evolutionary processes for a long time—ever since they began to breed better cereals or domestic animals. Even breaching the barriers between species is not new: since ancient times horses and donkeys have been crossed to produce mules. True, mules are sterile while gene splicing might lead to new creatures which are not; but all this shows, once again, the need for great caution. It would be one thing to engineer a new species, and other to release it upon the world.

Most genetically defective humans used to die in infancy. That may be regarded as the cruel wisdom of evolution. We interfere with this process when we use the latest medical technology to keep defective babies alive. Even treating diabetics with insulin, or prescribing spectacles for the short-sighted, prevents natural selection from reducing the prevalence of these conditions. Indeed, the entire system of social welfare that now exists in most developed countries is a huge interference with evolution: without it, the children of the poor would be less likely to survive and reproduce. Few people think this a sufficient reason for ending state assistance to the unemployed, single parents, orphans, and the disabled.

All this suggests that there is nothing sacred about the process of evolution. Evolution is not, after all, really wise. The application of such terms to the blind process of natural selection can only be a metaphor, and we should be careful not to be misled by it. Evolution does not minimize suffering. It cannot be relied upon to preserve the existence of our species or any other species. Humans can be wise or foolish: evolution can be neither.

When we first grasp the fact that the course of evolution is utterly indifferent to the well-being or ultimate fate of our species, we may leap to the conclusion that it is easy for us to use our intelligence to improve upon evolution. Perhaps we can; but it is unlikely to prove as straightforward as we first imagine. We should recall the early European settlers in Australia, who thought it would be easy to improve upon the natural environment by bringing over a few rabbits to add variety to the fauna, and some blackberries to provide food in the bush. We have now learnt, at immense cost, that the interrelatedness of our ecology makes it impossible to do just one thing—everything has an effect on something else. So too, when we try to improve upon evolution we may find that for some quite unexpected reason we have only made matters worse.

This is not an argument for prohibiting genetic engineering, but rather for putting a large warning label on it, and taking steps to ensure that the warning is heeded. We need to think about how genetic engineering might properly be used, and how it is to be controlled.

Therapeutics or eugenics?

We can distinguish two major purposes for genetic engineering in humans: to remove defects not present in normal members of the species (therapeutic genetic engineering); and to produce individuals with more desirable qualities than would be the case with normal reproduction (eugenic genetic engineering). Admittedly, the distinction is not clear-cut. We can all agree that sickle-cell anaemia is a genetic defect; but what about genetic factors that merely increase the probability of, say, suffering from heart-disease later in life? Genetic 'markers' that indicate such predispositions are now being discovered, and it seems that there are hundreds of them, covering a wide variety of diseases. Suppose that genetic engineering reached the point at which they could all be eliminated, thereby raising the expected life span of the 'corrected' individual from seventy-five years to ninety-five. Or what if the cause of ageing were discovered, and could be interfered with in such a way that youthful life, free of the diseases of degeneration, was possible indefinitely? Would this be thera-peutic or eugenic engineering?

Is this question merely semantic, or does some moral weight hang on the answer? Is therapeutic genetic engineering in a different moral category from eugenic? Many people believe it is. Remedying defects is at the core of medicine. Hence one may conclude that, as the President's Commission put it, 'the ethical and policy issues do not seem appreciably different from those involved in the development of any new diagnostic or therapeutic techniques'. There is no dispute about the initial judgement that, say, sickle-cell anaemia is a bad thing. If modern medicine can get rid of it, that will be good, just as getting rid of polio and smallpox were good. To get started on eugenic engineering, however, we need to decide which characteristics it is good to have to a higher than normal degree: intelligence? physical strength? altruism? drive? competitiveness? sensitivity of feeling? physical beauty? emotional toughness? The medical model is no help to us in sorting out these characteristics; hence we can agree on eliminating defects much more easily than we can agree on a moral basis for enhancing someone's genetic constitution above what would normally be expected.

There is some truth in this; but our example of the longer life-span that might be achievable by eliminating a range of genetic predispositions indicates that the picture is more complicated. To have twice the normal chance of a heart attack before the age of fifty is, we can all agree, a defect. The same can be said for a quadrupled risk of bladder cancer, or a 50 per cent greater chance of diabetes. Taken in itself, each predisposition is an abnormality. On the other hand to have no such predispositions at all is abnormal too—highly desirable as it may be. So while one might regard genetic engineering aimed at raising the expected life-span to ninety-five as an attempt at improving things beyond what is normal for our species, and thus as a form of eugenic engineering, this result might come about from eliminating a host of separate conditions. If we were to eliminate each of these conditions separately, we would clearly be doing therapeutic engineering.

Whatever we call it, this form of genetic engineering can be justified on the same basis as cases which are indisputably therapeutic. It does not matter whether the outcome is a life that is or is not better than the statistical norm; the essential element is that no one disputes that, other things being equal, it is better to live longer, in good health, than to die earlier. The acceptability of genetic engineering depends not on whether it falls under the label 'therapeutic' rather than 'eugenic', but on the ends towards which the engineering is directed. When the goal is something that would indisputably improve the human condition, safe and successful genetic engineering would be a good thing.

Again, however, there is a complication which should lead us to be cautious. Often the gene which predisposes to a disease also has some other, more attractive consequence—otherwise it would have been rapidly eliminated by natural selection. The gene for sickle-cell anaemia, for instance, is believed to confer greater immunity to malaria on those who are carriers. Hence carriers of this recessive gene are at an advantage in malaria-prone areas. This particular benefit has lost its value where malaria has been cleared up, or can be controlled by tablets. No one is going to oppose eliminating the disease on the grounds that this will also eliminate the benefit. But what are the benefits of other, less disastrous, genetic traits? If a certain type of genetic constitution is linked with a doubled chance of a heart attack, but is also associated with drive and ambition, is the benefit worth the risk? Is it possible that after eliminating all genetically-based above-average risks to health, we would find that we had inadvertently eliminated the characteristics that distinguish many of the most valued members of our species?

This difficulty illustrates two crucial points. The first is simply the need to proceed slowly and cautiously, under the watchful eye of an expert committee which can build up a body of information on the long-term outcome of individual attempts at genetic engineering. We shall say more about the need for this kind of committee shortly.

The second point is that, in seeking agreement on the goals to which genetic engineering should be directed, we must take into account possible costs as well as anticipated gains. There are two kinds of cases in which people will disagree about the net benefits of an attempt at genetic engineering. One is the case in which people disagree over the intrinsic desirability of the goal: is it good to have more people with IQs above 150? The other is the case in which an undisputed benefit, like a lowered risk of heart attack, must be balanced against what some see as a cost, like reduced drive. Since the two cases raise similar issues, we shall discuss only the former but our conclusions will be applicable to the latter type of case as well.

Goals and controls

It would be well to pause here and recognize that what we are talking about is different only in degree, and not in kind, from the human behaviour with which we are all familiar. The genetic constitution of our population is determined by human choices to a far greater extent than we like to admit. Whenever people choose one marriage partner rather than another, they affect the gene pool of the future. It would be foolish to deny that tall people often choose other tall people, particularly attractive people often choose others similarly fortunately endowed, sporting people often choose other sporting people, artistic people often choose other artistic people and so on. Sometimes we seek genetic consequences quite deliberately: when we make these choices of marriage partners we often have, decently interred at the back of our minds, the thought that a person with certain characteristics would make a good mother, or father, for our children. But even if this is the last thing in our minds when we choose our spouse, our choices will nevertheless determine the genetic constitution of the next generation.

What is new is the extent of the intervention that genetic engineering will make possible. The genetic lottery, which individuals have deliberately influenced since time began, will become a much less risky game of chance. To a far greater extent than ever before, the procreating generation will be able to determine the constitution of its successors. The question is: who should decide the genetic constitution of the next generation?

There is a central planning approach and a *laissez-faire* approach to handling disagreement over the desirability of a particular form of genetic engineering. The centralized approach would have the government, presumably acting through some expert committee, make the decisions. If the government considered high intelligence desirable, prospective parents would be offered the opportunity to have their embryos treated so as to raise the intelligence of the resulting child.

The government would, no doubt, find it difficult to get consensus on the qualities to be considered desirable, and that is one strong objection to this approach. A still more powerful reason against it, however, is that it puts a frightening amount of power into government hands.

To avoid this, one could take a 'free market' approach. Couples would make their own choices about the genetic constitution of their children. The problem of obtaining agreement about what is desirable is thus overcome, for agreement is unnecessary. All we need is tolerance of other people's choices for their own offspring. Individual freedom would be maximized, the State kept out, and the opportunities for misguided bureaucratic planning, or for something still more sinister, eliminated.

Neither the free market approach nor the central planning approach seems to us particularly satisfactory. The latter is far too much like Brave New World. Citizens should choose the constitution of their government; governments should not choose the constitutions of their citizens.

The free market approach is unsatisfactory for a different reason. It puts too much power in the hands of individuals who might use it irresponsibly or even pathologically. It is hard to imagine any parent using genetic engineering to produce a bodyguard of mindless clones, but it is just possible to imagine the sort of parents who might want to genetically engineer a nice, uniform football team.

We don't need to multiply instances to illustrate this point. There is, however, one aspect of individual choice in a competitive society that is worth noticing. If there is pressure on individuals to compete for status and material rewards, the qualities that give children a winning edge in this competition are not necessarily going to be the most socially desirable. For instance, above-average drive and ambition might make a child more likely to succeed—but too much striving for individual success will not make for a harmonious and co-operative society. Now consider the logic of leaving to individuals the choice of the type of children they will have. Suppose that genetic engineering has advanced to the stage at which we could significantly increase the drive and ambition of our children. Then any parents who wished their children to achieve high status and earnings would do well to make use of genetic engineering to produce an above-average level of drive and ambition. If many parents were to have such desires for their children, however, and to take the course that would give their children the best prospects of making it to the top, the result would simply be an increase in the average level of drive and ambition. Since this increase could do nothing to increase the number of winners—by definition, only a few can make it to the top—the result could only be greater frustration all round. So parents might try to engineer an even *greater* increase in drive and ambition for *their* children, thus leading to an upwards spiral in these characteristics which would be difficult to reverse. For although the increased emphasis on personal success might so reduce public-mindedness as to endanger the very existence of society as a communal enterprise, no parents could withdraw from this damaging spiral without condemning their own children to the lower ranks of the society. It would not be within the power of individuals to stop the accelerating rush to a society of supremely ambitious individualists. Such is the logic of rational self-interest—or family-interest—in a free-market situation.

Those still sceptical about the desirability of any State interference with individual choice in this area should remember that we are talking now of decisions that will (to a much greater degree than contemporary human procreation decisions) alter the public human environment. It is generally acknowledged that a society has the right to exclude certain types of people by the use of immigration laws. Some criteria of selection we do consider wrong—race is the obvious example—but selection on the basis of needed skills, or exclusion because of known criminal associations, is not considered objectionable. If a society is justified in thus selecting those who will become its members, surely it is also justified in excluding certain types of people which its own members are proposing to create.

Our suggestion therefore is this: the genetic endowment of children should be in the same hands it has always been in—the hands of parents. But parents who wished to use genetic engineering to bring about a characteristic which had not previously been sanctioned by the society through its government, should have to apply for permission. The public should know what such adventurous parents are proposing to do, and should equally have the right to say 'no'.

The machinery for such a system would not be too hard to devise. A broadly based government body could be set up to approve or reject particular parents' proposals for genetic engineering. It would consider whether the proposed piece of engineering would, if its practice became widespread, have harmful effects on individuals or society. If no harmful effects could be foreseen, the committee would license the procedure. This would mean that parents who wished to use it were free to do so. The committee would keep track of how many people were using each licensed procedure, and with what results. It could always withdraw a licence if unexpected harmful results emerged. Because the committee would need to agree only on the absence of harm, its deliberations would not be as difficult as they would be if agreement on positive benefit were required—though they would still be difficult enough.

The selective cloning of people with special abilities—an issue postponed from the previous chapter—could be handled in the same manner. In addition to keeping an eye on the problems of adjustment of the cloned individuals, the committee would also place strict limits on the number of clones that could be made from any one person, and on the extent of cloning in general. Thus a potentially harmful reduction of the diversity of the human gene pool could be avoided.

What concrete decisions might such a committee make, about the genetic engineering procedures it licensed and the individuals from whom cloning would be sanctioned? Presumably it would license proposals to increase intelligence (but cautiously, by small steps) and refuse to license proposals, if there were any, to diminish it. Presumably it would favour proposals which promoted the health of the future member of the society, and reject any that put it at risk. It might refuse to allow genetic engineering that would determine even for some positive characteristic (such as physical strength) if it was thought to be associated with some negative characteristic (such as propensity to heart attack). If it happened that scientists found genes associated with altruism or malice, it might license proposals to determine for the former, but not the latter. But what it should never do is make positive directions as to what should be done. It should confine itself to exercising the power of veto. In our view, choosing the positive content of the gene pool should remain the preserve of those who have always done it up until now—the parents.

Conclusion

8 HOW DO WE HANDLE THESE ISSUES?

A problem for democracy

We have looked at the revolution in human reproduction now taking place, and we have looked at what is coming. In this field future possibilities have a habit of turning into present realities before anyone is ready for them. When we began writing this book, pregnancies from donated embryos and pregnancies from frozen embryos were both mere future prospects: now as we draw the book to a close, they are realities. Though we are learning to expect the unexpected, it is not easy to predict what the next breakthrough will be, nor when it will come.

In this book we have suggested what should be done about the new ways of making babies. We believe that our conclusions are soundly based on a careful and dispassionate evaluation of all the relevant features of the case. If it were up to us, therefore, we would enact laws and regulations to give effect to the conclusions reached in the preceding chapters. Of course, it is not up to us; nor should it be. We are firm believers in democracy. We would like to see our conclusions adopted; but we want this to occur through discussion and rational persuasion rather than by dictatorial decree.

Unfortunately we can safely predict that our arguments will not convince everyone. To take one central example, we argued that the very early embryo is not yet a bearer of rights. Our arguments for this position are, as far as we can see, logically irrefutable. Yet we know from experience that many people presented with the argument remain unconvinced. Whatever the reason for our failure to convince, such disagreement raises fundamental issues both about the nature of ethics, and about the nature of democracy.

For ethics, the question raised is whether there is any objective truth about these matters. When we reach a basic difference in moral beliefs, must one side be irrational or in error? Or is it all just a matter of subjective attitudes, with any attitude being as defensible as any other, because ultimately where moral judgements are concerned there is no standard of truth or falsity? We shall return to these questions soon.

For democracy, the problem is how a government should deal with fundamental moral issues on which different sections of the community are deeply divided. All good democrats can accept the rights of different groups to practice their religion, express their beliefs, and live their lives in accordance with their own moral principles, in so far as these principles do not impinge upon the rights of others. But what is a government to do when it finds itself in a situation in which, whatever available option it chooses, there will be groups in the community who have a moral objection to that choice?

One dispute in which a government cannot avoid taking sides over is the funding of research. Suppose our government pays for a wide range of medical research, including research aimed at finding ways of overcoming infertility. It has, for example, sponsored research into the use of microsurgery to repair damaged Fallopian tubes. Now doctors come to ask for funds for research into a new and more promising method of enabling women with damaged tubes to have children: IVF. To develop this technique, the researchers propose to fertilize human eggs in the laboratory, grow the resulting embryos for a day or two, and then flatten them onto a glass slide for microscopic examination.

Should the government pay for such research? If it does, it will be acting contrary to the views of a substantial section of the community, who regard it as morally wrong to treat embryos in this manner. If it does not, it will be acting contrary to the views of another section of the community, who think the infertile should be helped and see nothing wrong with squashing sixteen-cell embryos.

In this situation pluralism and mutual tolerance are not enough. Those who want to experiment on human embryos may say that people with contrary views are perfectly free not to do such research, but should not impose their views on others. Those opposed to the experimentation, however, will argue that because the experimenters are asking for financial support from public revenue, it is they who are seeking to impose their views on taxpayers.

Moreover, even if the government should decide not to pay for the research, those who believe that embryos have rights will still not be satisfied. Consistently with their beliefs they may well go further and demand that privately funded research also be stopped, for they must hold that this, too, violates the rights of another—the embryo. Democratic pluralists may cherish the idea of people acting according to their different moral beliefs as long as they do not infringe the rights of others, but how can pluralism help when the question of whether an embryo counts as an 'other' is the very issue over which people differ?

If pluralism cannot provide a democratic solution to this difficulty, what about that other key democratic principle, majority rule? Should the government take some kind of referendum, and follow the views of the majority in allowing or disallowing the various procedures discussed in this book? That might be democratic, but it is not in keeping with the tradition of parliamentary democracy. In this tradition, the elected representatives of the public are not supposed simply to reflect the views of those who elect them. The classic statement is Edmund Burke's speech to his electors in Bristol: 'Your representative owes you, not his industry only, but his judgement; and he betrays instead of serving you if he sacrifices it to your opinion.'

The parliamentary tradition recognizes that electors will not have been fully informed on all issues, nor will they have had the time to give each issue the consideration it needs. If we think of representative democracy only as a device for expressing the views of the electorate, technical advances would have made it obsolete—we could all push buttons attached to our telephones to indicate what we thought about lower taxation, increased pensions, and bringing back the death penalty. The fact that we have not enthusiastically embraced these technical advances suggests that we do not equate 'democracy' with the enactment of whatever the majority thinks at any particular moment.

Ethics committees

The first reaction of democratic governments confronted with issues that raise awesome ethical dilemmas is more likely to be the appointment of a committee of inquiry than the holding of a referendum. In this way the government can bring in outside advice and expertise. No doubt some governments are also motivated by the thought that they may be able to defuse some of the controversy surrounding the issue by shunting it off to a non-political body, and then accepting the recommendations that body makes.

The first of these committees to look at some of the issues raised in this book was the Ethics Advisory Board of the United States Department of Health, Education and Welfare. In 1978 the Board agreed to review the ethical acceptability of research into IVF, so that the Department could decide whether to support a proposed research project on IVF. The Board reported in the following year, advising the Secretary for Health, Education and Welfare that research on IVF was ethically acceptable, under certain conditions. Four years later, the Secretary has still not acted on the Board's report. The unfortunate scientist whose research application led to the inquiry has since died, his application still pending.

Despite this inauspicious precedent, the British government has set up a Commission of Inquiry into IVF and related issues. The British Medical Association and the British Medical Research Council also have their own inquiries. In Australia, the States of Victoria, New South Wales, and Queensland now each have their own government-appointed committees looking into the matter. The Australian National Health and Medical Research Council has issued guide-lines allowing research on IVF, although not endorsing surrogate motherhood or cloning experiments.

Are these Boards, Commissions, and Committees the right way for democratic governments to handle these issues? Not everyone thinks so. After the United States Congress had set up a commission to conduct an investigation into 'the basic ethical principles which should underlie the conduct of biomedical and behavioural research', one critic, Ithiel de Sola Pool, condemned this as a task 'better suited to Iran's Revolutionary Council than to an American political commission'. Is Pool right to feel that deciding fundamental ethical questions may be the role of ayatollahs or priests in a theocracy, but is not a matter to be entrusted to a political commission in a pluralist democracy?

One ground for unease about the role of commissions may be that such commissions are usually seen as in some way 'expert'; yet once we drop the idea that ethical knowledge is to be gained by special insight into the will of God, it ceases to be at all clear what is involved in being an expert in ethics. When it comes to ethical judgements, isn't anyone's opinion as good as anyone else's?

The quest for consensus

One way of reconciling the objection to ethical expertise with the belief in the value of a committee of inquiry is to say that the purpose of setting up the committee is to bring together members of the different groups that make up a pluralist democracy, and see if they cannot find some common ground. In pursuit of this aim an American committee might be carefully chosen to include a Catholic, a Protestant, and a Jew, at lest two women and one black, and perhaps a businessman and a trade-unionist. But can such a committee really achieve a consensus view about any controversial ethical issue?

The answer is that it can—at a price. As an example, let us look at the already-mentioned report of the US Department of Health, Education and Welfare's Ethics Advisory Board. In particular, let us see how the Board managed to achieve consensus on the most fundamental moral issue it had to face: the moral status of the human embryo.

Since the research proposal that has led to the IVF inquiry involved fertilizing human eggs that were not to be transplanted into the womb, approving the research effectively meant approving of the disposal of early human embryos. It would scarcely seem possible for the Board to pass judgement on the propriety of this kind of research without taking sides on the issue that has dominated the highly charged debate over abortion: is human life sacrosanct from the moment of conception? Yet this is what the Board managed to do.

The Board began by recording its unanimous support for the

view that 'the human embryo is entitled to profound respect'. It then took back much of what this statement appeared to imply by adding: 'this respect does not necessarily encompass the full legal and moral rights attributed to persons'. In its conclusion it took back still more, for it found that research on *in vitro* fertilization, even without transfer of the embryo to the uterus, is 'acceptable from an ethical standpoint' provided certain conditions are met.

One is left wondering about the value of the 'profound respect' to which the Board believes the embryo is entitled. Clearly it does not prevent the deliberate creation of embryos that are doomed to destruction only a day or two after they are created. Does the profound respect in which they are to be held mean that they should be given a decent burial, instead of being tipped down the sink? The Board did not say.

When one reads the Board's own gloss on the meaning of the key phrase 'acceptable from an ethical standpoint' the recommendations become still murkier. The phrase does not mean, the Board says, 'clearly ethically right'; rather it means 'ethically defensible but still legitimately controverted'. In particular, the Board emphasized, the phrase does not mean that the ethical considerations against such research are insubstantial.

Put all that together and we have a masterpiece of consensus drafting. The human embryo is entitled to profound respect, but it is ethically acceptable to do research designed to create an embryo which will be watched for a short period and then disposed of; but then again, though this is 'ethically acceptable', it may still legitimately be controverted and the ethical considerations against it may well be substantial.

So pluralism and consensus are not incompatible—but this is scarcely an encouraging example. Nor was the final outcome any better. As we have seen, the Secretary for Health, Education and Welfare (then Joseph Califano) took no action on the report. This meant—and still means—that no government funds can be used for IVF research in the United States. Hence American scientists interested in developing IVF find themselves in the unfamiliar and uncongenial situation of having to stand by and watch their British and Australian counterparts making all the breakthroughs. Opponents of IVF are not happy either, however, because there is nothing to stop private clinics offering IVF to patients who can meet the cost. In practice IVF is going ahead in the United States without any government control.

That is one way an ethics committee can function in a democracy. Is it the only way? Might we not do better if we were a little less concerned about representing all the different groups in our pluralist society, and a little more ready to gather together those best qualified to consider the issues in an open and informed manner, unimpeded by adherence to sectarian doctrines which other members of society cannot be expected to accept? Is the idea of a committee of experts really so out of place in a democracy?

Ethical expertise and democracy

To answer this question we must first consider the extent to which there can be such a thing as an ethical expert. In most areas in which we accept a division between experts and those who are not experts, we can point to specific advantages which the experts have over the others. Expert mechanics know a lot about how cars work and what can be done to repair them when they go wrong. When my car won't start and I have exhausted my meagre list of remedies, expert mechanics can apply their superior knowledge to get my car running again. To distinguish expert mechanics from those who are not expert is therefore relatively straightforward (in theory). But what kind of superior knowledge do experts in ethics have, and how do we distinguish those who are expert from those who are not? I can tell when my car has been fixed properly, but how do we tell when our moral problems have been properly solved?

The question is not a simple one, and to answer it adequately would take us deeply into the nature of ethics. The question can be answered only on the premise that reason and logical argument have *some* role to play in ethics. If we abandon this premise, if we really accept that ethics is entirely a matter of subjective feelings or intuitions in which anyone's feelings are as good as anyone else's, then there really is no role for expertise in ethics. This is, however, an extreme view. Even those moral philosophers who call themselves subjectivists are ready to admit that subjectivism does not close the door on argument in ethics.

Obviously there is something wrong with—to give a crude example—claiming that all human life is equally valuable, and yet agreeing that a defective baby that contracts pneumonia should be left to die, when a normal baby would be given antibiotics. Thus subjectivism at the most fundamental level of ethics is still compatible with reason and argument playing a significant role in debates over ethical issues.

Once a role for reason and argument has been acknowledged, it follows that the first essential for an ethical expert is simply the ability that is required of all experts in any area that involves reason and argument—the ability to reason well and logically, to avoid errors in one's own arguments, and to detect fallacies when they occur in the arguments of others. These abilities are not, of course, limited to any small band of people with a specific kind of training. A training in philosophy tries to develop these abilities, perhaps more directly than most other forms of training, since it has logic as one of its branches; but a proper training in law, for example, would have similar aims, and there are some whose nose for a bad argument needs no training at all.

A second requirement for expertise is an understanding of the nature of ethics and the meanings of the moral concepts. Those who do not understand the terms they are using will do more to create confusion than to resolve controversies, and it is only too easy to become confused about the concepts used in ethics. A reasonable knowledge of the major ethical theories, such as utilitarianism, theories of justice and of rights, will also be useful. To decide ethical issues in a theoretical vacuum, without awareness of fundamental theories that bear on them, is not likely to be satisfactory in the long run. To adapt Santayana, those who do not know the work already done in their field are likely to waste a lot of time repeating it.

Finally, any kind of expert must be well informed about the facts of the matter under discussion. No one can be expert on a subject in medical ethics unless they know or are capable of learning the salient medical facts.

Looking back over these three points, two conclusions emerge. First, the idea of expertise in ethics does make sense. It is simply not the case that we are all equally good at detecting fallacious arguments, understanding moral concepts and theories, or grasping relevant facts—and all these skills contribute to what must be, by any standards, more soundly based ethical conclusions.

The second conclusion is that although ethical expertise exists, it is not limited to those who have very rare talents or special academic qualifications. Unlike, say, expertise in nuclear physics, expertise in ethics is open to any reasonably intelligent people who are prepared to put some time into gaining it. This means that democrats can recognize the existence of ethical expertise without thereby implying that all power should be put in the hands of a priesthood caste. On the contrary, a democrat will want to increase the level of expertise in the community so that there can be wider participation in the debate over ethical issues.

A National Bioethics Commission?

The revolution in reproduction has arrived. Governments all over the world now face the choice of regulating it, or leaving it to roll on, as the laws of supply and demand dictate.

We take a less alarmist view of these development than do many others. Nevertheless, we see a need for regulation in areas like surrogate motherhood, genetic engineering, and research on human embryos. Matters so momentous to a society as the manner in which its children are created should not be left to the more or less random outcome of individual decisions in a free-market situation. If these matters are to be regulated, however, it is not going to be good enough to set up short-term ethical committees which look at one particular problem, write a report, and then cease to exist. New issues are going to keep coming up, and they are serious enough to deserve a permanent body with the expertise needed to keep them under close watch.

The need for a permanent body is reinforced by the fact that the issues covered in this book, complex and far-reaching as they are, are only one set of the many different questions raised by new developments in medicine and the biological sciences. If we switch our attention to the opposite end of life, for example, we find another set of ethical problems generated by our new-found ability to keep alive, for indefinite periods, people whose quality of life is so low that they may be considered better off dead. Should such people be kept alive? If not, who decides when to turn off the machines? In most countries neither the law nor the ethical codes of medical practitioners give clear answers.

We propose a permanent organization—we shall refer to it as a National Bioethics Commission—with the staff and resources to make recommendations on all these issues. In every country this would take a slightly different form. In Australia, for example, it could be set up very inexpensively and effectively as a standing committee of the Law Reform Commission. Stimulating public debate would be part of the brief of such a Commission. The role of this debate would be to ensure that all the information and arguments came out into the open: the Commission would not be aiming at accommodating all points of view in its final recommendations, since, as we have seen, some views are mutually contradictory. On the contrary, sometimes the Commission might have to challenge widely held but ill-founded moral beliefs. It cannot do this if consensus is its aim.

While not striving for consensus at the level of its specific recommendations, the Commission should base its recommendations on general ethical principles that all can accept. It should not appeal to revelations of God's commands, to the idea that our natural capacities, for instance our sexuality, were 'given' to us for specified purposes, nor to belief in the existence of an immortal soul. To base recommendations on such doctrines would preclude their rational acceptance by members of the community who did not share these beliefs. We all agree on enough basic ethical principles to make it unnecessary to prejudice the argument with such controversial assumptions.

Instead the Commission should look to general principles which depend on no sectarian allegiances. What will lead to the kind of society in which the greatest possible number are able to satisfy their most important needs and desires? What will most reduce misery and suffering? These are basic moral principles that all of us can accept, at least as an important part of morality. To see their validity, all we have to do is think about the significance our own needs and desires have for us, and then apply the Golden Rule, so that we allow to others as much significance for their needs and desires as we would have them allow to ours. The outcome of this kind of 'universalizing' of our own needs and desires is a concern for the welfare of everyone.

To this fundamental principle of social welfare the Commission may wish to add, in the appropriate cases, constraints based on justice, equality, and rights. Reasonable people may differ on the importance of these principles and the extent to which they should be taken into account. What matters in the long run, however, is not that there be unanimity for each recommendation, but that standards of argument be developed which make it possible for anyone to follow the Commission's reasoning and either accept its recommendations, or show where it has gone wrong. This is the only kind of consensus that is worth while: not consensus that uses lofty meaningless rhetoric to paper over deep divisions, but consensus built on respect for the role of reason and argument in reaching conclusions.

If a Bioethics Commission were to have some prospect of success in this task, its members would have to be selected because of their expertise and their ability to think clearly and without fixed preconceptions. We should not expect that every section of the community would be represented. When we set up an expert committee to look into the nation's energy requirements, we don't insist on having a Catholic, a Protestant, a Jew, a black, and a woman on the committee. We have independent standards of expertise in this area, and we want the best possible committee for the job. If there is such a thing as expertise in ethics, the same principles should apply. It is, in any case, political window-dressing rather than real pluralism that produces such carefully contrived membership lists. Does anyone really believe that the female point of view, or the black point of view, or even the Catholic point of view, is so universally accepted by all members of each group that it can be represented by one person?

Would an expert Bioethics Commission be undemocratic? We think not. Since the government of the day could always reject its recommendations, the democratic system would control the Commission, rather than the other way around. Of course, the idea would be that the government did *not* reject its recommendations; but this would be because the recommendations would be so carefully and sensibly defended by the Commission that the government would be persuaded. There is nothing undemocratic about the power of rational argument.

We would like to conclude our book on this confident note; but in all honesty we cannot do it. If, over the last few pages we have waxed lyrical over the virtues of expert commissions, it is not because we believe they hold all the right answers to the problems that confront us. In any area, committees of experts can make mistakes. Sometimes the mistakes are horrendous. The Bioethics Commission we have proposed would also, no doubt, make mistakes. We expect only that it would make fewer mistakes than any alternative method of tackling the very difficult issues with which it would deal. Moreover, even as it made its mistakes, it would be contributing to the task of educating itself, and the community as a whole, in how to think about the future. We will need to learn fast.

APPENDIX 1
Reports and Statements

A. Ethics Advisory Board, US Department of Health, Education and Welfare, *Report and Conclusions: HEW Support of Research Involving Human* In Vitro *Fertilization and Embryo Transfer*, 4 May 1979 (extract)

Chapter VI Summary and conclusions

It is now technically possible to fertilize a human egg outside the body of a woman and then transfer the fertilized egg (sometimes called a blastocyst or preimplantation embryo) back into the woman to establish a pregnancy. For some women, *in vitro* fertilization may be the only way to bear children of their own. It does not appear, however, that the procedure for achieving pregnancy by this means is yet very effective; the best available data indicate that a number of attempts have been necessary before a pregnancy in a particular woman can be established, if at all. In addition, many questions remain as to the safety of the procedure for the offspring. Nevertheless, there is reason to believe that clinics may soon be established, both in this country and abroad, where *in vitro* fertilization and embryo transfer will be offered as 'therapy' for infertile couples.

The Board is required by HEW regulations to review research proposals involving human *in vitro* fertilization and advise the Secretary as to their 'acceptability from an ethical standpoint'.[1] This phrase is broad enough to include at least two interpretations: (1) 'Clearly ethically right' or (2) 'ethically defensible but still legitimately controverted'. In finding that research involving human *in vitro* fertilization is 'acceptable from an ethical standpoint' the Board is using the phrase in the second sense; the Board wishes to emphasize that it is *not* finding that the ethical considerations against such research are insubstantial. Indeed, concerns regarding the moral status of the embryo and the potential long-range consequences of this research were among the most difficult that confronted the Board.

In its deliberations on human *in vitro* fertilization, the Board confronted many ethical, scientific and legal issues. Among the more difficult were the following: (A) The moral status of the embryo; (B) the safety and efficacy[2] of the procedure; (C) the potential long-range adverse effects of such research; and (D) the appropriateness of Departmental support.

A. After much analysis and discussion regarding both scientific data and the moral status of the embryo, the Board is in agreement that the human embryo is entitled to profound respect; but this respect does not necessarily encompass the full legal and moral rights attributed to persons. In addition, the Board noted the high rate of embryo loss that occurs in the natural process of reproduction. It concluded that some embryo loss associated with attempts to assist otherwise infertile couples to bear children of their own through *in vitro* fertilization be regarded as acceptable from an ethical standpoint, under certain conditions, as more fully described below.

B. The Board is concerned about still unanswered questions of safety for both mother and offspring of *in vitro* fertilization and embryo transfer; it is concerned, as well, about the physical and mental health of the children born following such a procedure and about their legal status. Many women have told the Board that in order to bear a child of their own they will submit to whatever risks are involved. The Board believes that while the Department should not interfere with such reproductive decisions, it has a legitimate interest in developing and disseminating information regarding safety and health so that fully informed choices about reproduction can be made.

C. A number of fears have been expressed with regard to adverse effects of technological intervention in the reproductive process: fears that such intervention might lead to genetic manipulation or encourage casual experimentation with human embryos, or bring with it the use of surrogate mothers, cloning, or the creation of genetic hybrids. Some have suggested that such research might also have a dehumanizing effect on investigators, the families involved, and society generally. (See Chapter III of this report.)

Although the Board recognizes that there is an opportunity for abuse in the application of this technology as other technologies, it concluded that a broad prohibition of research involving human *in vitro* fertilization is neither justified nor wise. Among the developments warned against by some who testified before the Board, a few (*e.g.*, the cloning of human beings and the creation of animal/human hybrids) are of uncertain or remote risk. Other possible developments, such as the use of surrogate mothers, may be contained by regulation or legislation. Other abuses may be avoided by the use of good judgment based upon accurate information of the type collected by the Board and now being disseminated in this report. Finally, where reproductive decisions are concerned, it is important to guard against unwarranted governmental intrusion into personal and marital privacy.

D. The question of Federal support of research involving human *in vitro* fertilization and embryo transfer was troublesome for the Board in view of the uncertain risks, the dangers of abuse and because funding the procedure is morally objectionable to many. In weighing these considerations, the Board noted that the procedures may soon be in use in the private sector and that Departmental involvement might help to resolve questions of risk and avoid abuse by encouraging well-designed research by qualified scientists. Such involvement might also help to shape the use of the procedures through regulation and by example. The Board concluded that it should not advise the Department on the level of Federal support, if any, of such research; but it concluded that Federal support, if decided upon after due consideration of all that is at issue, would be acceptable from an ethical standpoint.

Evidence presented to the Board indicates that human *in vitro* fertilization and embryo transfer techniques may, in the near future, be employed throughout the world in both research and clinical practice settings. The Board believes that data from these activities as well as related types of animal research should be collected, analyzed and, when appropriate, given wide public dissemination. Accordingly, the Board recommends in conclusion #4 below, that the Department take the primary initiative in carrying out these functions.

Having carefully weighed diverse ethical points of view and a broad base of scientific considerations regarding human *in vitro* fertilization and embryo transfer, the Board has concluded that: (1) The Department should consider support of more animal research in order to assess the risks to both mother and offspring associated with the procedures; (2) the conduct of research involving human *in vitro* fertilization designed to establish the safety and effectiveness of the procedure is ethically acceptable under certain conditions; (3) Departmental support of such research would be acceptable from an ethical standpoint, although the Board did not address the question of the level of funding, if any, which such research might be given; (4) the Department should take the initiative in collecting, analyzing and disseminating data from both research and clinical practice involving *in vitro* fertilization throughout the world; and (5) model or uniform laws should be developed to define the rights and responsibilities of all parties involved in such activities.

Finally, the Board is aware of the possibility of research that involves the collection and culture of early human embryos in the laboratory which have been fertilized naturally rather than *in vitro*. The ethical aspects of such research, which appears to bear a close resemblance to research involving *in vitro* fertilization, have not been examined by the Board. Therefore it has not reached a conclusion concerning the ethical acceptability of these procedures. However, the Board intends to consider in the near future the need for setting standards for such research.

Conclusion (1). The department should consider support of carefully designed research involving *in vitro* fertilization and embryo transfer in animals, including nonhuman primates, in order to obtain a better understanding of the process of fertilization, implantation and embryo development, to assess the risks to both mother and offspring associated with such procedures, and to improve the efficacy of the procedure.

Discussion: As indicated in Chapter III of the Board's report, available scientific data do not indicate clearly either the relative safety or the efficacy of procedures of *in vitro* fertilization and embryo transfer. Some scientists have suggested that *in vitro* fertilization may result in a higher incidence of abnormal embryos than is associated with the normal reproductive process, although there are no animal data that clearly demonstrate such an effect. Neither are there data that demonstrate an absence of increased abnormality in embryos following *in vitro* fertilization. The Board feels that additional data should be gathered that might indicate whether abnormal embryos are more likely to result and, if so, whether there is a significant increase in the risk of abnormal offspring actually being born following such procedures.

Experts appearing before the Board agreed that there has been insufficient controlled animal research designed to determine the long-range effects of *in vitro* fertilization and embryo transfer. The lack of primate work is particularly noteworthy in view of the opportunity provided by primate models for assessing subtle neurological cognitive and developmental effects of such procedures. The Board has been advised that controlled studies of embryo transfer following *in vitro* fertilization in animals, designed to include developmental assessments, may be feasible and may permit more confident estimates of the risk to human offspring associated with such procedures.

Information regarding the effectiveness of the procedures for *in vitro* fertilization and embryo transfer is also lacking. It does not appear possible to predict with reliability the number of laparoscopies and embryo transfers that might be required, or the likelihood of success of the procedures for any couple, given the fact that, to date, only three successes have been reported in humans and that very limited information is available concerning this work. Such data as are available suggest that any woman hoping to bear a child through *in vitro* fertilization is likely to face numerous unsuccessful procedures and delays with no assurance of achieving her goal.

Careful research with animal models might provide a more accurate estimate of the chances of achieving a successful pregnancy. It might also reduce the inconvenience and risk to women of undergoing multiple procedures to establish a pregnancy by improving techniques for recovering ova, identifying embryonic abnormalities and achieving implantation. It is often the case in medicine that, even after therapies are already being applied to humans, investigations continue in animals in order to test further or to improve their safety and effectiveness. The

Board believes that the Department should consider support of well-designed animal studies whether or not human research or clinical trials are also in progress.

Conclusion (2). The Ethics Advisory Board finds that it is acceptable from an ethical standpoint to undertake research involving human *in vitro* fertilization and embryo transfer provided that:

A. If the research involves human *in vitro* fertilization without embryo transfer, the following conditions are satisfied:

1. The research complies with all appropriate provisions of the regulations governing research with human subjects (45 CFR 46);

2. The research is designed primarily: (A) To establish the safety and efficacy of embryo transfer and (B) to obtain important scientific information toward that end not reasonably attainable by other means;

3. Human gametes used in such research will be obtained exclusively from persons who have been informed of the nature and purpose of the research in which such materials will be used and have specifically consented to such use;

4. No embryos will be sustained *in vitro* beyond the stage normally associated with the completion of implantation (14 days after fertilization); and

5. All interested parties and the general public will be advised if evidence begins to show that the procedure entails risks of abnormal offspring higher than those associated with natural human reproduction.

B. In addition, if the research involves embryo transfer following human *in vitro* fertilization, embryo transfer will be attempted only with gametes obtained from lawfully married couples.

Discussion: This conclusion relates to the ethics of conducting research involving *in vitro* fertilization in general; it does not address the question of Departmental support of such research. The purpose of this more general conclusion is to provide guidance to Institutional Review Boards and other groups who were asked to review research that will not be supported by HEW.[3] Whether or not the Department decides to provide funds for such research, the Board wishes to express its views regarding the conduct of human *in vitro* fertilization and embryo transfer, so that review groups may benefit from the deliberations of the Board as they conduct their own review of specific research proposals.

As emphasized above, the Board believes that much remains to be learned about the safety and effectiveness of these procedures before they can be considered standard, accepted medical practice. Research designed to provide reliable data regarding safety and efficacy is acceptable from an ethical standpoint if conducted within the constraints indicated above. In the case of research involving embryo transfer, the Board intends not only that the gametes be obtained from lawfully married couples but also that the embryo be transferred back to the wife whose ova were used for fertilization.

The Board also discussed research designed primarily to establish safety and efficacy but which may, in addition, obtain information of scientific importance unrelated to *in vitro* fertilization and embryo transfer. The Board believes that such research, if performed as a corollary to research designed primarily to establish safety and efficacy of *in vitro* fertilization and embryo transfer, would also be acceptable from an ethical standpoint.

Conclusion (3). The Board finds it acceptable from an ethical standpoint for the department to support or conduct research involving *in vitro* fertilization and embryo transfer, provided that the applicable conditions set forth in conclusion (2) are met. However, the Board has decided not to address the question of the level of funding, if any, which such research might be given.

Discussion: 1. *Departmental support*. The Board consciously adopted the language 'acceptable from an ethical standpoint' to indicate the limits of its inquiry. Even though the members are aware that ethical considerations pervade decisions regarding the level, if any, of Departmental support of human *in vitro* fertilization, the Board has concluded that it lacks the resources needed to render meaningful advice with respect to such decisions. The Board, therefore, defers to established political, scientific and administrative procedures for allocating public research funds.

The Board wishes to note that such decisions have significant ethical dimensions. For example, some believe that research involving human *in vitro* fertilization should have a relatively low priority at a time when other health needs, arguably more basic in character and long-term in nature, are unmet. Others find such research objectionable either on grounds related to the moral status of the embryo or because it may lead to undesirable genetic interventions or have a long-range adverse effect. (See Chapter III of this report.) Still others believe that research on human *in vitro* fertilization and embryo transfer should have a high priority because it might help parents overcome physical obstacles to having their own children and ensure the mothers' safety and the normality of offspring.

The Board has found that these and other ethical arguments for and against public funding of research involving human *in vitro* fertilization, by themselves, are not conclusive. Instead, the Board believes that the questions of whether to fund and at what level should be made in the larger context where all relevant data and arguments—scientific, political, economic, legal and ethical—can be considered. In that context questions such as health and safety, availability of funds, and alternative research proposals, must be considered along with the very difficult type of ethical issues described above which arise in allocation of resources.

2. *Research without embryo transfer.* As previously noted the risks of producing abnormal offspring are still undetermined; therefore, an important goal would be to gain as much information as possible from well-designed research on *in vitro* fertilization not involving embryo transfer in humans. The Department should conduct a careful scientific evaluation of the possibility, supported by some expert testimony before the Board, that animal research and studies involving human *in vitro* fertilization without embryo transfer, over a relatively short period, might substantially increase our knowledge concerning the possible risk of abnormal offspring as well as lead to the development of safe and more effective techniques.

3. *Research involving embryo transfer.* While initial research efforts designed to gain as much information as possible from animal studies and human research not involving embryo transfer may

be desirable, the Board does not wish to discourage planning and preparation that may lead to clinical trials or other forms of research involving embryo transfer. The Department's participation in, or support of, clinical trials is often an effective method to evaluate the safety and efficacy of innovative medical procedures, particularly as the use of the procedures increases.

4. *Research for other purposes*. Potentially valuable information about reproductive biology, the etiology of birth defects, and other subjects may be revealed through research involving human *in vitro* fertilization without embryo transfer, and unrelated to the safety and efficacy of procedures for overcoming infertility. The Board makes no judgment at this time regarding the ethical acceptability of such research nor does it speculate about what research might be sufficiently compelling to justify the use of human embryos. Instead, it notes that applications for support of such research should be submitted to the Board for ethical review in accordance with 45 CFR 46.204(d).

5. *Pending Research Application*. Given the criteria specified in Conclusion (2) and incorporated in Conclusion (3) for evaluating research involving human *in vitro* fertilization, and the Board's views about Departmental support of such research, the Board recommends that the Secretary refer the pending application of Vanderbilt University back to the National Institutes of Health for a determination as to whether the proposal meets those criteria and for further review in light of the considerations set forth in this report.

Conclusion (4). The National Institute of Child Health and Human Development (NICHD) and other appropriate agencies should work with professional societies, foreign governments and international organizations to collect, analyze and disseminate information derived from research (in both animals and humans) and clinical experience throughout the world involving *in vitro* fertilization and embryo transfer.

Discussion: The Board is aware that the most valuable information regarding *in vitro* fertilization and embryo transfer is likely to come from well-controlled clinical trials. But it is expected that *in vitro* fertilization and embryo transfer will soon be performed in clinics throughout the world, sometimes without benefit of research design or experimental controls. It would be unfortunate not to have access to the information that might be gained from such clinical experience, notwithstanding the fact that well-designed investigations would be preferable. With that in mind, the Board recommends that every effort be made to collect whatever information may be elicited from practitioners in this country and abroad. NICHD should also consider suggesting to practitioners a basic protocol for collecting vital information, to which each would be encouraged to add their own observations.

The data from such clinical experience and from research conducted throughout the world should be analyzed along with that derived from animal studies so that individuals contemplating *in vitro* fertilization and embryo transfer will have access to the best information available regarding risks to both mother and offspring. Timely dissemination of the information would increase the opportunity for investigators, clinicians and prospective patients to be fully informed.

Conclusion (5). The secretary should encourage the development of a uniform or model law to clarify the legal status of children born as a result of *in vitro* fertilization and embryo transfer. To the extent that funds may be necessary to develop such legislation, the department should consider providing appropriate support.

Discussion: The Board is concerned about the ambiguity regarding the legal status of children born following artificial insemination and a similar ambiguity that may surround the legal status of children born following *in vitro* fertilization and embryo transfer. The Board is also concerned about lack of clarity regarding the legal responsibilities of those who utilize, support, or permit use of such procedures. Because of the complexity of the legal problems involved in new techniques for human reproduction, the Board recommends that a model or uniform law be drafted that would establish with clarity the rights and responsibilities of donor and recipient 'parents', of offspring and of those who participate in the process of reproduction through new technologies.

The Board urges that such a uniform or model law be drafted by the National Conference of Commissioners on Uniform State

Laws, the American Law Institute, or some other qualified body. Because of the complex nature of the subject matter, however, the Board is aware that the task may be a major undertaking and suggests that the Department consider providing funds for drafting the legislation. Since the purpose is to safeguard the health and welfare of children and their families, it appears to be an appropriate project for Departmental support.

Notes
1. 45 CFR 46.204(d).
2. By 'efficacy' the Board means not only whether the procedure can be done but also how efficient it is, *e.g.*, the number of procedures required to achieve the desired result.
3. Federal law requires all institutions receiving research funds from HEW to establish an Institutional Review Board (IRB) to review biomedical and behavioral research involving human subjects (Pub. L. 93–348). The Department, in implementing that law, requires all such research conducted at an institution to be reviewed by the IRB, whether or not the research is supported by HEW.

> From *Federal Register*, 18 June 1979, pp. 35033–35058. The Ethics Advisory Board was chaired by James C. Gaither, a San Francisco attorney.

B. National Health and Medical Research Council, Australia, *Statement on In Vitro Fertilization and Embryo Transfer* (Supplementary Note 4 to *Statement on Human Experimentation*, 3 September 1982)

In vitro fertilization (IVF) of human ova with human sperm and transfer of the early embryo to the human uterus (embryo transfer, ET) can be a justifiable means of treating infertility. While IVF and ET is an established procedure, much research remains to be done and the NH & MRC Statement on Human Experimentation should continue to apply to all work in this field.

Particular matters that need to be taken into account when ethical aspects are being considered follow.

(1) Every centre or institution offering an IVF and ET program should have all aspects of the program approved by an

institutional ethics committee. The institutional ethics committee should ensure that a register is kept of all attempts made at securing pregnancies by these techniques. The register should include details of parentage, the medical aspects of treatment cycles, and a record of success or failure with:

  (i) ovum recovery;
  (ii) fertilization;
  (iii) cleavage;
  (iv) embryo transfer; and
  (v) pregnancy outcome.

These institutional registers, as medical records, should be confidential. Summaries for statistical purposes, including details of any congenital abnormalities among offspring, should be available for collation by a national body.

(2) Although IVF and ET as techniques have an experimental component, the clinical indications for their use, treatment of infertility within an accepted family relationship, are well established. IVF and ET will normally involve the ova and sperm of the partners.

(3) An ovum from a female partner may either be unavailable or unsuitable (e.g. severe genetic disease) for fertilization. In such a situation the following restrictions should apply to ovum donation for embryo transfer to that woman.

  (a) the transfer should be part of treatment within an accepted family relationship;
  (b) the recipient couple should intend to accept the duties and obligations of parenthood;
  (c) consent should be obtained from the donor and the recipient couple;
  (d) there should be no element of commerce between the donor and recipient couple.

(4) A woman could produce a child for an infertile couple from ova and sperm derived from that couple. Because of current inability to determine or define motherhood in this context, this situation is not yet capable of ethical resolution.

(5) Research with sperm, ova or fertilized ova has been and remains inseparable from the development of safe and effective IVF and ET; as part of this research other important scientific

information concerning human reproductive biology may emerge. However continuation of embryonic development in vitro beyond the stage at which implantation would normally occur is not acceptable.

(6) Sperm and ova produced for IVF should be considered to belong to the respective donors. The wishes of the donors regarding the use, storage and ultimate disposal of the sperm, ova and resultant embryos should be ascertained and as far as is possible respected by the institution. In the case of the embryos, the donors' joint directions (or the directions of a single surviving donor) should be observed; in the event of disagreement between the donors the institution should be in a position to make decisions.

(7) Storage of human embryos may carry biological and social risks. Storage for transfer should be restricted to early, undifferentiated embryos. Although it may be possible technically to store such embryos indefinitely, time limits for storage should be set in every case. In defining these time limits account should be taken both of the wishes of the donors and of a set upper limit, which would be of the order of ten years, but which should not be beyond the time of conventional reproductive need or competence of the female donor.

(8) Cloning experiments designed to produce from human tissues viable or potentially viable offspring that are multiple and genetically identical are ethically unacceptable.

(9) In this as in other experimental fields those who conscientiously object to research projects or therapeutic programs conducted by institutions that employ them should not be obliged to participate in those projects or programs to which they object, nor should they be put at a disadvantage because of their objection.

C. Victorian Government Committee to Consider the Social, Ethical and Legal Issues Arising from In Vitro Fertilization, *Interim Report*, September 1982 (extract)

---

5. *The most common situation*

5.1. The history and present practice of IVF in Victoria

constitute the context in which the Committee has begun its work. It has considered a large number of papers and submissions dealing with IVF. It is aware that there is strong support for and substantial opposition to the process.

5.2. In its Interim Report the Committee has not considered a number of issues relating to IVF which it has identified, which it believes deserve careful attention and about which it expects to make particular recommendations.

5.3. 'Some of these issues are of great urgency, in that they involve parts of IVF programmes which are already being carried out or have been plainly foreshadowed in Victoria. These are freezing and storage of embryos and the use of donor ova and donor sperm. Other issues have been raised.

5.3.1. These include surrogate motherhood, that is, implantation of an embryo in the uterus of a woman who is not the contributor of the ovum or oocyte.

5.3.2. Fertilization of embryos specifically for research and experimentation or for therapeutic use.

5.4. Other issues, which may be described as more contentious include cloning, development of hybrids and other genetic engineering techniques—either for research and experimentation or therapeutic use. Finally, there is the possibility of IVF followed by laboratory nurture and birth—the 'test-tube baby' complete.

5.5. In its Interim Report the Committee has concentrated its attention solely on the most common situation in which IVF is employed in Victoria. This involves a husband and wife supplying their own genetic material for the production of an embryo or embryos which will be inserted into the uterus of the wife with the aim of implantation occurring and a successful pregnancy ensuing.

5.6. *The Committee considers this form of the procedure to be acceptable to the Victorian community and accordingly recommends that it be recognized in those terms.*

5.7. In reaching this conclusion, the Committee acknowledges that, in the Victorian community, there are several groups who, while expressing strong support and sympathy for infertile couples, reject IVF as unnatural conception. Others reject it because of inadequate prior research on animals, of the inherent experimentation on and risk of damage to the embryos produced, and of the possible risk of personality traumas in the children as they develop through childhood and adolescence to adulthood.

While developments since the first successful IVF birth have tended to diminish but not dispel some of these concerns, the first remains. Associated with this is a deeply held philosophical view that the embryo is, immediately after fertilization, a form of human life to which both protection and respect must be accorded. (The level and strength of that recognition and protection, in terms of legal rules conferring it, is itself a matter of debate.) The Committee recognizes, therefore, that some groups in the Victorian community will not participate in or countenance IVF. Their views deserve respect, in line with the views of members of the community who oppose other lawful procedures well established in current medical practice. But, nonetheless, the practice of IVF in the most common situation does, in the Committee's view, command substantial support in the Victorian community.

5.8. *Safeguards.* Even in what it believes to be the most common situation in which IVF is employed it is the Committee's view that the above-mentioned matters require safeguards to protect the interests of the community and the individuals involved in the programme, including the embryo formed in the laboratory.

5.8.1. *Centres conducting IVF and embryo transfer.* It will be apparent from the contents of section 4 of this report that the process of IVF is a complicated one requiring skilled doctors, technicians and support staff. The procedure is a relatively expensive one. The Committee has concluded, therefore, that IVF should only be conducted in hospitals authorized to do so by, and responsible to, the Health Commission of Victoria. It recommends that legislation to give effect to this recommendation be enacted as soon as possible. The terms of any authorization should encompass some of the matters considered in succeeding paragraphs.

5.8.2. *Counselling.* The Committee is concerned about the needs and the wishes of infertile couples who seek to resolve the problems that may ensue from their infertility. In this connection it notes that it is misleading to describe IVF and ET as a cure or even a treatment of infertility. It is rather a *means* of circumventing infertility and, for this reason, may even tend to discourage couples involved in a programme from facing up to the anger, guilt, despair and isolation that, to a greater or lesser degree, go together with the knowledge that they are infertile. For this reason the Committee believes that counselling must be available in any IVF programme.

The Committee further believes that counsellors should be specifically trained to deal with the problems of infertility. Counselling available in any IVF programme shall include:

5.8.2.1. provision of general information about an IVF programme and what it may involve for the couple;

5.8.2.2. support for the couple while on the waiting list, when involved in the programme, and, if pregnancy is not achieved, for 12 months after leaving the programme; and

5.8.2.3. infertility counselling which may, if necessary and mutually agreed, take the form of therapeutic counselling.

Adoption of this recommendation should help to ensure that infertile couples arrive at a position from which they can determine for themselves whether or not to become and remain involved in an IVF programme. A counselling programme should from the outset provide information about self-help groups.

5.8.3. *Information and Consent.* The Committee believes that each couple seeking admission to an IVF programme must be provided with clear and comprehensive information about the programme. Each couple must be advised of any risks involved in the programme and of its likely duration and given the most accurate information about the prospects of success. This will then permit each couple to express in writing their free and informed consent to participate in the programme.

5.8.4. *Community Education.* Some of the problems encountered by infertile couples stem in part from community ignorance concerning the extent and nature of infertility. The Committee has therefore decided that provision should be made for appropriate forms of education in secondary schools and in other suitable contexts, including the media, with the aim of increasing the awareness and the understanding of infertility in the Victorian community. This should include information about the causes of infertility, about methods to prevent its occurrence, about treatments which may be available, about adoption, and about marriage without children. The Committee has been impressed by the work done and the publications produced on this subject by the Institute of Family Studies and the Citizens Welfare Service of Victoria.

5.8.5. *Selection of Participants.* In the context of the Interim Report the Committee is of the view that the procedure should be available, at present, only to married couples. While there is increasing tolerance of and some recognition of de facto relationships in the community, it is in the context of a husband/wife relationship and the framework of the traditional family that the community in general approves of IVF.

The Committee believes that the selection of couples for the IVF programme should not be solely made on the basis of first in line or the capacity to pay, but should be made on the basis of defined priorities relating to individual needs. In view of the cost of the programme, the complexity of the techniques used, and the large number of patients seeking treatment, each couple should have attempted other appropriate means of treatment prior to selection for the IVF programme. Where infertility has proven unresponsive to other means of treatment or the couple has sought alternative treatment for a period in excess of 12 months then such couple shall be entitled to be selected to join the IVF programme if they are otherwise suitable candidates for treatment. Information relating to alternative means of treatment should be widely disseminated.

5.8.6. *Surplus Embryos.* The Committee appreciates the deep concern of a section of the Victorian community which considers that from the moment of fertilization an embryo is a human being to be accorded a substantial measure of respect and rights (some would say at the same level as persons born alive). At the same time the Committee is aware that not all sections of the community share this philosophical view of personhood and the attitude towards embryonic life that derives from it. In these circumstances, and for the purpose of the Interim Report, the Committee is of the view that in the Victorian community IVF and ET are acceptable if *all* fertilized oocytes are transferred to the uterus of the mother.

A majority of the Committee also believes that where a couple requests that attempts be made to fertilize all oocytes recovered, and where too many embryos are produced for all to be transferred, the wishes of the couple concerning handling of such excess embryos should be respected. The majority opinion takes into account data indicating a higher rate of successful pregnancies when all oocytes recovered are fertilized. This view is not held by the Chairman, the Reverend Dr. Harman and Mrs. Hay who are of the view that the problem of surplus embryos needs to be further considered in depth.

Three members of the Committee, the Chairman, Reverend Dr. Harman and Mrs. Hay believe that until the Committee has had time to consider fully the implications of alternatives such as freeze thawing of embryos, donation of embryos, and surrogate motherhood, that these procedures should not be employed in IVF programmes in Victoria. The remaining members believe the process of freeze thawing should be allowed to continue while this is being considered.

5.9. *Legal Implications in the Most Common Situation.* The Committee considers that in the most common situation there are no questions of status which arise specifically out of IVF procedures. The Committee believes that the legal status of the child born as a result of IVF in that situation is clear; it is the legitimate issue of the marriage.

The Committee has not considered questions of criminal responsibility or civil liability which may arise in the context of IVF.

The Committee is aware that the Standing Committee of Attorneys-General has been considering the preparation of legislation in relation to the legal status of children born as a result of artificial insemination by donor (AID) and IVF. The Committee supports the view that there should be uniform legislation on this subject, and would value the opportunity to examine the draft legislation, with a view to considering its substance and its form in connection with its further work.

5.10. *Recommendations.* In view of the matters considered above, the Committee recommends that, pending its further report or reports, the Government should:

5.10.1. institute a campaign of public education on the nature, causes and treatment of infertility.

5.10.2. enact legislation to authorize hospitals as centres in which IVF programmes may be conducted. The terms of the authorization should provide that:

— before a couple is admitted to the IVF programme they must have undertaken all other medical procedures during a period in excess of 12 moths which may, in their particular circumstances, overcome their infertility;

— the IVF programme be limited to cases in which the gametes are obtained from husband and wife and the embryos are transferred into the uterus of the wife;

— admission to the IVF programme is preceded, accompanied and followed by appropriate counselling.

Published by the Committee, which was chaired by Professor L. Waller, Victorian Law Reform Commissioner.

D. Victorian Government Committee to Consider the Social, Ethical and Legal Issues Arising from In Vitro Fertilization, *Report on Donor Gametes in IVF*, August 1983 (extract)

6. Summary of recommendations

6.1. The use of donor sperm in IVF should be permitted in the Victorian community.

6.2. The use of donor ova in IVF should be permitted in the Victorian community.

6.3. The Government should initiate a programme of information about the causes and incidence of infertility, with special attention to those aspects which have led to the development of AID programmes, and the use of donor sperm in IVF programmes, and the proposed use of donor ova.

6.4. The matters set out in para. 6.3 should be incorporated into an appropriate course of study prescribed for secondary schools students.

6.5. Comprehensive information, including ethical, social, psychological and legal matters bearing on all aspects of the treatment of infertility, should be available for all infertile couples.

6.6. The information described in para. 6.5 should be translated into as many community languages as possible.

6.7. Counselling should precede, accompany, and follow participation in donor gametes in IVF programmes.

6.8. Consent to the use of donor gametes in IVF should be given, and recorded in a document, by the couple before they begin to participate in the procedures. A copy of the consent document should be given to the partners, and the original retained by the hospital.

6.9. Before a couple is admitted to an IVF programme involving the use of donor gametes they should have undertaken all other appropriate medical procedures, during a period in excess of 12 months, which may, in their particular circumstances, overcome their infertility.

6.10. Admission to a donor gametes in IVF programme should be based on the criterion of need, taking into account not only medical but also social and psychological considerations.

6.11. Admission to a donor gametes in IVF programme should not disqualify patients from admission to or retention on adoption waiting lists.

6.12. Donors of gametes should not receive payment.

6.13. Donations of gametes from children should be prohibited.

6.14. Selection of donors should be based not only on medical but also on social and psychological considerations.

6.15. Donors should receive comprehensive information and counselling about the implications of gametes donation.

6.16. Donors should complete and sign a document consenting to the use of the donated gametes, and no recovery of gametes should be undertaken before the completion of that document.

6.17. Donors of gametes may withdraw consent before the donated gametes have been used in an IVF programme.

6.18. The use of known donors in donor gametes in IVF programmes should be permitted, where both partners request it. Special counselling should be provided for the donors and the couple.

6.19. It should be unlawful to seek or use donor ova obtained from women in an IVF programme unless consent has been given before the treatment has been instituted.

6.20. The hospital should offer non-identifying information about the sperm or ovum donor to the recipient.

6.21. The hospital should offer non-identifying information about the recipients to the gametes donor.

6.22. The hospital should advise the donor, if the donor so chooses, of the results, in the form of non-identifying information, of any successful use of the gametes donated.

6.23. The Health Commission should establish a central registry containing comprehensive information about donors whose gametes have been successfully used in an IVF programme.

6.24. Each hospital authorized to conduct an IVF programme using donor gametes should maintain its own register of all donors whose gametes are used, and should transmit regularly to the Health Commission details of the pregnancies resulting from the successful use of donor gametes.

6.25. Information in the central registry should be exempt from the provisions of the *Freedom of Information Act* 1982.

6.26. It should be unlawful to use donor gametes in IVF in such a way as to confuse those concerned about the genetic background of any child born.

6.27. Hospitals should be specifically authorized to use donor gametes in IVF programmes.

6.28. The terms of the authorization should provide that conscientious objection to participation by doctors and other personnel in the hospital shall be recognized.

6.29. The provisions of the draft *Artificial Conception Bill* 1983 should be amended to make it clear that they apply to children born as a result of the use of donor sperm in IVF, as well as those born as a result of AID procedures.

6.30. The draft Bill should be amended to provide for the status of children born as a result of the use of donor ova in IVF, in terms which copy those provisions for children born as a result of the use of donor sperm.

6.31. The use of donor embryos in IVF should be permitted in the Victorian community.

6.32. It should be unlawful for donor embryos to be used except in the case of couples whose infertility cannot be overcome by other means, or where the couple may transmit undesirable hereditary disorders.

6.33. Information and counselling, where appropriate, should draw attention to the complexities that may arise from the use of donor embryos in IVF.

6.34. Donors' gametes should not be used to create donor embryos unless each donor has given explicit written consent to such use.

6.35. When more than one embryo is transferred at the same time it should be unlawful for the embryo to be derived from more than one male or more than one female donor.

Published by the Committee, which was chaired by Professor L. Waller.

E. Statement by the Medical Research Council (UK), 'Research related to human fertilization and embryology'

Introduction

The purpose of this statement is to set out the principles which the Medical Research Council believe should guide those whose research involves the use of in vitro fertilisation with human gametes. The council's intention is that the guidance should be followed by workers supported by the council, but the principles are believed to be generally valid for all such research.

Background

In 1978 the council set up an advisory group to review policy on research related to in vitro fertilisation and embryo transfer in humans. The group decided to concern itself only with the ethics of such work and did not examine specific scientific aspects. The group advised the council that scientifically sound research involving in vitro fertilisation—where there was no intent to transfer the embryo to the uterus—should be allowed to proceed if its aim were clearly defined and acceptable; and concluded that, in the context of female infertility due to tubal occlusion, in vitro fertilisation with subsequent embryo transfer should be regarded as a therapeutic procedure covered by the normal ethics of the doctor/patient relationship. The council endorsed these views.

In May 1982 the advisory group was reconvened with an expanded membership and terms of reference as follows:

'to consider recent and potential developments in research related to human fertilisation and embryology, and to advise the council on these and on the ethical grounds they should take into account in considering research proposals in these areas'.

The group's further conclusions have been accepted by the council as an appropriate basis for MRC policy.

Guidelines for research related to human fertilisation and embryology

(i) Scientifically sound research involving experiments on the processes and products of in vitro fertilisation between human gametes is ethically acceptable and should be allowed to proceed on condition both that there is no intent to transfer to the uterus any embryo resulting from or used in such experiments and also that the aim of the research is clearly defined and directly relevant to clinical problems such as contraception or the differential diagnosis and treatment of infertility and inherited diseases.

(ii) Informed consent to research involving human ova or sperm should be obtained in every case from the donor(s); sperm from sperm banks should not be used unless collected and preserved specifically for a research purpose. Approval for each experiment should be obtained from the appropriate scientific and local ethical committees.

(iii) When human ova have been obtained and fertilised in vitro for a therapeutic purpose and are no longer required for that purpose it would be ethical to use them for soundly based research provided that the informed consent of both donors was obtained.

(iv) Human ova fertilised with human sperm should not be cultured in vitro beyond the implantation stage; and should not be stored for unspecified research use.

(v) Although it is not always possible to extrapolate results from animal work to the human situation, studies of animal gametes and embryos are useful to elucidate the potential risks of in vitro fertilisation and embryo transfer. Tests of animal embryos in appropriate animal models are necesary before it can be assumed that freezing and storage of the embryo does not cause harm to the conceptus.

(vi) Studies on interspecies fertilisation are valuable in providing information on the penetration capacity and chromosome complement of sperm from subfertile males, and should be supported. The fertilised ova should not be allowed to develop beyond the early cleavage stage.

From the *British Medical Journal*, 285 (20 November 1982), p. 1480. The MRC Advisory Group was chaired by Professor G. S. Dawes of the Nuffield Institute for Medical Research, Oxford.

F. British Medical Association working group on in vitro fertilisation and embryo replacement and transfer, *Interim report on human in vitro fertilisation and embryo replacement and transfer*

(1) The working group on in vitro fertilisation was set up by the council of the BMA in March 1982 and council approved the following terms of reference in May 1982:

'To consider ethical guidance to the medical profession on the current programme of in vitro fertilisation in the United Kingdom, and the social and ethical implications of the future application of this work and other related techniques that may be derived from it in relation to medical practice.'

(2) Certain forms of human infertility arise from defects, anatomical or otherwise, which impede or obstruct the normal processes by which an ovum shed at ovulation is fertilised by sperm and the resultant fertilised ovum (embryo) passes to the uterus and implants permitting development of the embryo in the majority of instances. Other forms of human infertility include oligospermia and unexplained infertility. The use of donor sperm or donor ova may be desirable when one or other members of the couple have a transmittable genetic defect. In vitro fertilisation embodies medical techniques designed to overcome such problems.

(3) These in vitro fertilisation techniques involve the removal from the woman by a surgical operation, usually a laparoscopy, of one or more ova at the phase of impending bursting of the Graafian follicle. The Graafian follicle may have reached this stage naturally, but sometimes procedures inducing ovulation or superovulation are instituted and the latter may lead to more than one 'ripe' ovum being available for harvesting. Each ovum is then maintained in an artificial environment and is shortly bathed in vitro in the sperm of the male partner of the couple. If fertilisation occurs and early cell divisions of the embryo are initiated, the embryo is replaced in the woman's uterus via the cervix after which implantation may take place and development of the embryo may proceed to full term and to a live birth.

(4) The techniques of in vitro fertilisation and embryo replacement are new and are still developing. In the most successful centres at the present time, only about one in five in

vitro fertilisations and embryo replacements leads to an established pregnancy, and the miscarriage rate is about 25%, somewhat higher than normal. Therefore, these procedures should be carried out only in a few special centres in the United Kingdom, each providing the necessary special medical and back up scientific expertise supported by appropriate facilities, clinical and otherwise.

(5) It is important that each centre should have a system for recording all attempts to secure pregnancy and the outcomes thereof. As with medical records, such in vitro fertilisation registers at centres would be confidential but numerical summaries for statistical purposes, together with details of any congenital abnormalities among the offspring, should be available for collation by a central body to which all viable births following in vitro fertilisation and embryo replacement should be notified. The central body should be the Health Departments, which, under the direct control of the chief medical officers, would hold the confidential central registers. The chief medical officers would be notified of all viable births, and details such as congenital abnormalities. (Among the known 128 live births following in vitro fertilisation and embryo replacement one case of a cardiac abnormality in a twin in Australia has been reported.)

(6) The treatment of infertility by in vitro fertilisation and embryo replacement should be preceded by assessment of the stability of the family relationship of the couple concerned and of the sincerity of their intention to accept the duties and obligations of parenthood.

(7) As laparoscopy and the other procedures of in vitro fertilisation and embryo replacement, which are not without risks, may have to be repeated on a number of occasions in the attempts to establish a pregnancy leading to a live birth, it is important that the couple should fully understand, and be robust enough to meet, these demands which may fall particularly heavily on the woman of the couple and which may come to a disappointing end without the achievement of a live birth.

(8) It is ethically acceptable to undertake in vitro fertilisation using the sperm and ova of the couple concerned with subsequent replacement in the uterus of the woman of the couple.

(9) Given informed consent by all parties concerned, the use of

donated sperm for in vitro fertilisation of the ovum of the female partner with embryo replacement in her uterus or the use of a donated ovum for in vitro fertilisation by the male partner's sperm with embryo transfer to the female partner is not unethical. In the rare cases in which neither party can produce viable gametes (sperm or ova), the use of donated sperm and donated ova for in vitro fertilisation and transfer to the female member of the couple may be ethically acceptable.

(10) It is proper and important that appropriate steps should be taken to ensure that effectiveness of in vitro fertilisation and embryo replacement and transfer treatments are maximised and risks minimised. To this end the observation of fertilised ova in excess of those needed for embryo replacement or transfer will add to medical knowledge and may yield important information not otherwise obtainable, for instance, optimising of the in vitro nutrient media for in vitro fertilisation for the developing embryo or establishing the genetic make up of such embryos sibling to that which was used for embryo replacement. Such observations should normally be completed within five to 10 days and always within a maximum of 14 days of fertilisation of the ovum by in vitro fertilisation. The donors' wishes in relation to the ultimate disposal should, as far as possible, be respected.

(11) The endometrium of a woman in whom superovulation has been induced for harvesting of multiple ova may not be in the ideal state for implantation of an in vitro fertilisation embryo. If observations showed that embryos within a few days of in vitro fertilisation could be stored without damage—for example, by freezing—and then unfrozen later for successive superovulation so that the embryo replacement could be synchronised to the optimal endometrial conditions for implantation, then the woman of the couple might be spared the multiple procedures and laparoscopies which may be required at the present time in the repeated attempts to achieve a live birth. (Storage should not exceed 12 months, and the couple's wishes in relation to ultimate disposal should, as far as possible, be respected.)

(12) It is envisaged that centres are likely to be within a university teaching hospital complex and that proposed programmes of observations on fertilized ova in excess of those

needed for embryo replacement should be approved by the local ethical committee.

(13) The working group has yet to be satisfied that to undertake in vitro fertilization with the sperm and the ova of a couple and to transfer the embryo to the uterus of another woman who might carry the embryo to term on behalf of the couple will ever be acceptable. (The term 'surrogate motherhood' has been applied to this situation and is distinct from the situation described in paragraph 9 above.)

(14) It is not ethically acceptable for medical practitioners to be involved in in vitro fertilisation and embryo replacement procedures in which the gametes (sperm or ova), embryos, or parts thereof are subjected to manipulations, including procedures designed to change their genetic make up or to induce the formation of multiple progeny ('cloning'), if there is any intent to transfer the resulting embryos to a uterus.

(15) The Medical Research Council has made a statement on 'Research related to human fertilisation and embryology' (20 November 1982, p 1480). The BMA working group concurs with the guidance given in that statement by the Medical Research Council and draws the attention of the medical profession to the statement.

(16) The BMA working group intends to review the ethical guidance offered above (including that on the duration of storage given in paragraph 11) in the light of the observations made, as in vitro fertilisation, embryo transfer, and other related techniques develop.

Addendum: Artificial insemination from a donor

(1) Although artificial insemination from a donor is not within the formal remit of the working group on in vitro fertilisation, the group makes the comments below as relevant to its deliberations.

(2) Artificial insemination from a donor has been used for many years in some cases of infertility as an accepted medical practice. The working group is informed that the birth of a child as a result of artificial insemination from a donor is usually registered by a parent with the registrar for births and deaths as if that child were the natural child of the couple. Although such an act of registration appears contrary to English law, such

registrations appear to be condoned as part of the present social scene.

(3) It is the view of the working group that the law should be changed so as to dispel any ambiguity of the legal status of a child born as a result of artificial insemination from a donor. Some states—for example, in North America—are reported to have made such provision.

(4) In 1973 following the deliberations of a panel set up by the BMA under the chairmanship of Sir John Peel, the BMA recommended legitimation for the artificial insemination from a donor child and stressed the need for procedural and personal safeguards at law for the parties concerned. The BMA's central ethical committee in 1979 reaffirmed this view and as a result the annual representative meeting passed the following resolution:

'That this meeting supports council's efforts to secure a change in the law, so that a child born as a result of artificial insemination from a donor to which the husband of the mother has consented in writing is recognised as legitimate from the time of confirmation of conception.'

(5) The BMA working party on in vitro fertilisation commends this view and hopes eventually that the Law Commission (subsequent to the tentative proposals made in its working paper No 74) will make appropriate recommendations. It also hopes that such recommendations will lead to a reform of the law by a draft Bill to be placed before parliament.

(6) The working group noted that changes in the law in connection with artificial insemination from a donor might also provide protection in the analogous field of ovum donation.

From the *British Medical Journal*, 286 (14 May 1983), pp. 1594–5. The BMA working group was chaired by Professor J. P. Quilliam, St Bartholomew's Hospital Medical College, London.

APPENDIX 2

IVF Patients and Their Attitudes to Ethical Issues: Replies to a Questionnaire

by Patsy Littlejohn, School of Social Work, Phillip Institute of Technology, Bundoora, Victoria

The questionnaire was distributed to couples on the IVF Programme at the Queen Victoria Medical Centre, Melbourne, during the period October to December, 1982.

Method of distribution
Questionnaires were distributed by hand to couples when they attended the hospital for treatment.

Return of questionnaires
Respondents were supplied with a self-addressed, postage-paid envelope and requested to return the completed questionnaire within one week.

Number of questionnaires distributed
300 (150 couples)

Response
114 questionnaires returned: 53 couples
                                       1 male
                                       7 female

Analysis of data
Data was coded for the computer and analysed using the Statistical Package for Social Sciences (SPSS).

A summary is presented of the information obtained from the questionnaires on the respondents and their answers to selected questions.

Note
In the expression 'n =' which appears in some of the following tables, 'n' refers to the number of respondents to whom the question applied.

Where the expression does not appear, the question applied to all respondents, i.e. n = 114.

1. Respondents

Age

Years	25–30	31–35	36–40	41–45	Over 45	Not answered
%	19.3	36.8	25.5	13.1	0.9	4.4

Nationality

	%
Australian	74.6
Naturalized Australian	16.7
Other: British	5.2
United States	1.7
Maltese	0.9
New Zealand	0.9

Occupation

	Men n = 54 %	Women n = 60 %	Men & women n = 114 %
Not working	3.7	30.0	17.5
Professional	33.3	25.0	28.9
Managerial	11.1	0	5.3
Clerical	13.0	21.7	17.5
Skilled	24.1	8.3	15.8
Semi-skilled	11.1	8.3	9.6
Unskilled	3.7	1.7	2.6
Student	0	5.0	2.6

Education

	%
Secondary level only	44.7
Trade qualification	18.4
Tertiary degree & higher	36.9

Religion

Denomination	%
Catholic	21.9
Church of England	20.2
Presbyterian/Uniting	9.6
Other Christian	4.4
Jewish	2.6
No church	41.2

	Yes %	No %	Not answered %
Q. Would you describe yourself as a religious person?	36.0	63.1	0.9
Q. Do you belong to any church	57.9	41.2	0.9

	Often %	Some-times %	Rarely %	Never %	Not answered %
Q. When you have decisions to make in your everyday life are you influenced in your decisions by what your church says you ought to do?	5.3	8.8	18.4	65.8	1.8

Children

Important reasons for wanting children

	No. of respondents indicating an important reason	Percentage total respondents
Having children was the reason you married.	12	10.5
Your spouse wants a child.	65	57.0
To carry on the family name and inheritance.	14	12.3
A child is important for a happy marriage.	16	14.0
To prove you are able to have a child.	6	5.3
Life is not complete unless you have children.	34	29.8
Pressure from your parents.	1	0.9
Pressure from your friends.	0	0
You think you would be a good parent.	50	43.9
Your friends have children.	6	5.3
You feel selfish without a child.	5	4.4
You feel useless without a child.	13	11.4
All women should experience pregnancy and birth.	19	16.7
You have a strong desire to have a child.	92	80.7

Q. Would you use the following alternatives for having a family?

	Yes %	No %	Undecided %	Not answered %
Adopt a normal Australian baby?	63.2	34.2	–	2.6
Adopt a handicapped baby?	7.0	79.8	1.8	11.4
Adopt a handicapped older child?	3.5	83.3	0.9	12.3
Adopt a child from a poor Asian country?	36.0	55.3	0.9	7.9
Accept an embryo transfer from another IVF couple?	54.4	38.6	0.9	6.1
Accept an embryo transfer when a donor egg is used, fertilized by husband's sperm?	72.8	21.9	–	5.3
Use a 'surrogate mother' to grow your own IVF embryo?	28.1	66.7	1.8	3.5
Artificial insemination by donor (AID)?	57.0	39.5	–	3.5

IVF programme

Q. How long have you been on the IVF waiting-list?

Months							
6–12	13–18	19–24	25–30	31–36	37–42	43–48	Not answered
% 12.3	37.7	26.3	5.3	7.0	0	3.5	7.9

Q. How many IVF treatment cycles have you attempted?

	0	1	2	3	4	5	6	7
%	26.3	38.6	10.5	14.9	5.3	2.6	0	1.8

	Yes %	No %	Parents deceased %	Some %	Not answered %
Q. Do you have any children?	20.2	78.9			0.9
Q. Have you told your parents you are on an IVF programme	80.7	13.2	2.6		3.5
Q. Have you told all members of your family you are on an IVF programme?	59.6	34.2			6.1
Q. Have you told your close friends you are on an IVF programme?	77.2	18.4			4.4
Q. Have you told all your friends you are on an IVF programme?	22.8	64.9		0.9	11.4
Q. Have you told your work colleagues you are on an IVF programme?	35.1	55.3		1.8	7.9

	Yes %	No %	Not answered %
Q. Do you think all costs should be rebatable as with other medical costs?	93.0	6.1	0.9

Q. If you were no longer able to claim expenses on health insurance would you be able to afford to remain on the programme?

Not at all %	For only one treatment %	For a limited number of treatments %	Money is no barrier %	Not answered %
7.0	12.3	64.9	14.9	0.9

In-vitro fertilization and embryo transfer

Q. Do you think IVF children should be told that they were conceived *in vitro*?

Yes %	No %	Uncertain %	Not important %	Not answered %
77.2	15.8	2.6	0.9	3.5

Q. Do you think the following should be admitted to IVF programmes?

	Yes %	No %	Uncertain %	Not answered %
Married couples without any children.	99.1	–	–	0.9
Married couples with only one child.	93.0	2.6	1.8	2.6
Married couples with two or more children.	36.0	58.8	1.8	3.5
Couples who are not married but have a stable *de facto* relationship without any children.	62.3	33.3	0.9	3.5
Couples who are not married but have a stable *de facto* relationship with only one child.	53.5	43.0	–	3.5
Couples who are not married but have a stable *de facto* relationship with two or more children.	22.8	73.7	–	3.5
Any couple who asks for it.	14.0	77.2	2.6	6.1
Women without a current male partner (donor sperm would be used).	19.3	73.7	2.6	4.4
Lesbians or other women not wishing to have a sexual relationship with a man.	14.9	78.9	2.6	3.5

3. Eggs and sperm

Q. If fertility drugs lead to multiple eggs being produced how many eggs should be collected?

Not more than three %	More than three %	All that are available %	Not answered %
2.6	11.4	83.1	0.9

	Yes %	No %	Unsure %	Not answered %
Q. Do you approve of using donor sperm in IVF when the husband's sperm is unsuitable?	75.4	12.3	0.9	11.4
Q. If several eggs are collected do you think they all should be inseminated?	64.0	33.3	1.8	0.9
Q. If not all eggs are inseminated do you think it is all right if the other eggs are:				
(i) Frozen and stored for your use later?	93.0	4.4	–	2.6
(ii) Frozen and made available for donation?	78.9	11.4	–	9.6
(iii) Made available for donation straight away?	76.3	14.0	–	9.6
(iv) Discarded?	18.4	63.2	1.8	16.7

4. Embryos

Q. Who should make decisions regarding the use of IVF embryos?

The couple alone	The IVF team in consultation with the couple	The IVF team alone
%	%	%
18.4	79.0	2.6

Q. If an embryo has been frozen and one of the couple dies who should make decisions regarding use of the embryo?

The remaining spouse	The IVF team in consultation with the remaining spouse	The IVF team alone
%	%	%
25.5	71.9	2.6

	Yes %	No %	Unsure %	Not answered %
Q. Do you think it is all right if any embryos not transferred back into the egg donor following IVF are:				
(i) Discarded?	33.3	58.8	–	7.9
(ii) Frozen and stored for later transfer to the egg donor?	88.6	4.4	–	7.0
(iii) Frozen and donated to another woman at a later date?	73.7	14.9	–	11.4
(iv) Donated immediately to another woman?	76.3	18.4	–	5.3
(v) Used for research?	68.4	23.7	0.9	7.0
Q. Do you consider any embryos created from the egg and sperm of you and your partner are the property of you and your partner?	90.4	7.9	–	1.8
Q. If an IVF couple should separate or divorce should the consent of both partners be obtained for the use of any embryos?	82.5	10.5	–	7.0
Q. If both members of the IVF couple should die who should make decisions about the use of any frozen embryos?				
(i) The IVF team.	67.5	21.1	–	11.4
(ii) Discard all frozen embryos.	24.6	50.0	–	25.4

5. General aspects

	Yes %	No %	Unsure %	Not answered %
Q. Do you feel adequately informed on all the IVF procedures carried out?	85.1	14.9	–	–
Q. Are you worried that IVF and embryo transfer procedures may result in an abnormal child?	23.7	76.3	–	–
Q. Would you agree to a termination of pregnancy if tests indicated the foetus was abnormal?	80.7	9.6	3.5	6.1
Q. Do you think further experiments should be done on 'spare' embryos to gain more information if this information will help to produce normal pregnancies?	81.6	17.5	0.9	
Q. Would you approve of 'spare' embryos being grown in the laboratory to obtain material which might have medical uses?	36.0	24.6	0.9	38.6
Q. Would you approve of 'spare' embryos being used in cloning experiments?	6.1	52.6	0.9	40.4
Q. Would you approve of 'spare' embryos being used in genetic engineering procedures to remove any defect or diseases present in the embryo?	43.9	17.5	0.9	37.7

	Yes %	No %	Unsure %	Not answered %
Q. Would you like the scientists to be able to select the sex of the embryo before transfer?	26.3	71.9	–	1.8
Q. Do you think work should be done on developing the embryo totally outside the body? If this is possible, do you think it is desirable?	14.0	74.6	3.5	7.9
Q. Should IVF couples be able to sell their embryos?	0.9	97.4	–	1.8
Q. Would you approve of a woman selling her eggs?	3.5	93.9	0.9	1.8
Q. Do you approve of a man selling his sperm?	7.0	91.2	–	1.8

6. Surrogate mothers

	Yes %	No %	Unsure %	Not answered %
Q. Should surrogate mothers be allowed if the genetic parents cannot have a child in any other way?	78.1	17.5	–	4.4
Q. Should surrogate mothers be allowed if the genetic parents could have a child in the ordinary way but prefer not to become pregnant?	1.8	93.0	–	5.3

	Yes	No	Unsure	Not answered
	%	%	%	%
Q. Should surrogate mothers be able to charge for their services?	54.4	34.2	0.9	10.5
Q. If surrogate mothers are able to charge for their services, should it be a set fee?	54.4	19.3	0.9	25.4
Q. If surrogate mothers are able to charge for their services, should they be able to charge whatever people are prepared to pay?	15.8	43.0	0.9	40.4
Q. If a surrogate mother wishes to keep the baby should she have the right to do so?	14.9	74.6	1.8	8.8

NOTES ON SOURCES

1 Fertilization outside the body

14–16 Edwards and Steptoe describe how they pioneered IVF in Robert Edwards and Patrick Steptoe, *A Matter of Life* (Sphere, London, 1981). A brief account of the Australian work is in Carl Wood and Ann Westmore, *Test-Tube Conception* (Hill of Content, Melbourne, 1983) pp. 41–8.

17 Grobstein used the term 'external fertilization' in his book, *From Chance to Purpose: An Appraisal of External Human Fertilization* (Addison-Wesley, Reading, Mass., 1981).

17–20 The experiences of Jan and Len Brennan are drawn from two sources. One is an article by Peter Roberts entitled 'The Brennan Story: A small miracle of creation', which was first published in *The Age* (Melbourne) and has been reprinted in William Walters and Peter Singer (eds.), *Test-Tube Babies* (Oxford University Press, Melbourne, 1982). The other source is two talks given by the Brennans to a Monash University Centre for Human Bioethics conference. These talks have been published as 'Case Study: Becoming IVF Parents' in Margaret Brumby (ed.), *In Vitro Fertilization: Problems and Possibilities* (Monash University Centre for Human Bioethics, Melbourne, 1982), pp. 12–16.

20–2 Isabel Bainbridge wrote of her experiences in 'With Child in Mind', in Walters and Singer (eds.), *Test-Tube Babies*, pp. 119–27. This account was supplemented by an interview with Isabel and Toby Bainbridge. The quotations are taken from the interview and subsequent correspondence.

23 On the loss of embryos in normal pregnancy, see Carl Wood and Ann Westmore, *Test-Tube Conception*, pp. 98–9. For Edwards's suggestion that IVF might eventually reach a higher success rate than natural reproduction, see 'What now for test-tube babies?', *New Scientist*, 4 February 1982, p. 313.

24 For the discussion of success rates we are indebted to 'External (In Vitro) Human Fertilization: A Five-Year Assessment of a New Reproductive Technology', an unpublished paper by Clifford Grobstein

Michael Flower, and John Mendeloff. A short version has been published as 'External Human Fertilization: An Evaluation of Policy', *Science*, 222 (14 October 1983), pp. 127–33. See also *Test-Tube Conception*, pp. 94–6.

25 The success rate following transfer of more than one embryo is taken from Alan Trounson, Carl Wood, and John Leeton, 'Freezing of Embryos', *Medical Journal of Australia*, 2 October 1902, pp. 332–3. The 'births per created embryo' figures were supplied by Dr Alan Trounson in a personal communication.

26–7 For estimates of infertility, see the paper by Grobstein, Flower, and Mendeloff, cited above. The quotation from Dr Georgeanna Jones comes from *New Scientist*, 4 February 1982, p. 313.

28 The cost of IVF in Australia is analysed by the Victorian Government Committee to Consider the Social, Ethical and Legal Issues Arising from In Vitro Fertilization, in its *Interim Report* (September 1982). United States costs are set out in the paper by Grobstein, Flower, and Mendeloff.

30 The estimate of total US spending on medical research is taken from a statement by Dr Andrew Rowan made at hearings before the Subcommittee on Science, Research and Technology of the Committee on Science and Technology of the US House of Representatives, 13–14 October 1981, published by the US Govt Printing Office, Washington, 1982, p. 300. The figure for the Australian National Health and Medical Research Council is provided in the Council's publication, *Medical Research Projects, 1981* (Australian Government Printing Service, Canberra, 1982).

31–2 The US public opinion polls were commissioned by the Ethics Advisory Board of the Department of Health, Education and Welfare, and the results published in sections 21–2 of the *Appendix* to its report, *HEW Support of Research Involving Human In Vitro Fertilization and Embryo Transfer* (US Govt Printing Office, Washington, DC, 4 May 1979).

32–4 Full details of the Australian and British polls were kindly made available by the Roy Morgan Research Centre, Melbourne. For the British poll, see also *The Times* (London), 11 October 1982, and for the most recent Australian poll, *The Bulletin* (Sydney), 17 May 1983. See also M. Brumby, 'Australian Community Attitudes to *In Vitro* Fertilization', *Medical Journal of Australia* 2, no. 12 (1983), pp. 650–3.

2 IVF: The simple case

35 The *Interim Report* of the Victorian Government Committee to

consider the Social, Ethical and Legal Issues Arising from In Vitro Fertilization was published by the Committee in September 1982. Its conclusions dealing with 'the simple case' are reprinted in Appendix 1 of this book.

36 Mill's essay 'Nature' is included in J. S. Mill, *Three Essays on Religion* (Longmans, London, 3rd ed. 1885).

40 See Pope Paul VI, *Humanae Vitae: On the Regulation of Birth* (Paulist Press, New York, 1968). For discussions of contraception and natural law by Roman Catholic writers, see Germain Grisez, *Contraception and the Natural Law* (Bruce Publishing Co., Milwaukee, 1964) and John Finnis, 'Natural Law and Unnatural Acts', *Heythrop Journal*, 11 (1970) pp. 365–87.

41 The passage is quoted from Fletcher's article, 'Ethical Aspects of Genetic Controls', *New England Journal of Medicine*, 285 (1971), p. 781.

42 This passage is from Ted Howard and Jeremy Rifkin, *Who Should Play God?* (Dell, New York, 1980), p. 206.

45 Kass's arguments are to be found in *HEW Support of Research Involving Human In Vitro Fertilization and Embryo Transfer, Appendix*, section 2. The quotations are from pp. 21 and 32. The reply by Gorovitz is section 3 of the *Appendix* to the HEW report, and the quotation is from p. 12 of that section. Grobstein's comments are on p. 71 of *From Chance to Purpose*.

46–7 For a lively account of the 1971 Washington symposium, see Edwards and Steptoe, *A Matter of Life*, pp. 123–6. Paul Ramsey's article, 'Shall we "Reproduce"?' appeared in *Journal of The American Medical Association*, 220 (1972), pp. 1346–50 and 1480–5; Leon Kass's 'Making Babies: The New Biology and the "Old" Morality' was published in *The Public Interest*, 26 (1972), pp. 18–56. The study by the US National Research Council appeared under the title *Assessing Biomedical Technologies: An Inquiry into the Nature of the Process* (National Academy of Sciences, Washington, DC, 1975). Edwards's confidence in the absence of 'intermediates' is expressed in *A Matter of Life*, p. 111.

47 Details of the Del Zio case are given in Thomas Carney, *Instant Evolution* (University of Notre Dame Press, Notre Dame, 1980), p. 107; the full legal citation of the case is *Del Zio v. Presbyterian Hospital*, 1974, Civ 3588 (S.D.N.Y. 1978).

48 The remarks by Michael Thomas were quoted in *New Scientist*, 4 February 1982, p. 315. See also J. Schlesselman, 'How Does One Assess the Risk of Abnormalities from Human *In Vitro* Fertilization?',

Appendix to the HEW Report, section 17, and also in *American Journal of Obstetrics and Gynaecology*, 135 (1979), pp. 135–48.

49 Laurence Fitzgerald's article 'Test Tube Morality in the Final Analysis' is from *The Advocate* (Melbourne), 5 April 1982. The statement by the Roman Catholic Bishops of Victoria is in the same newspaper, 19 August 1982.

52–4 The quotations are from Pius XII's 'Address to the Catholic Union of Midwives', 29 October 1951, available in O. M. Leibhard (ed.), *Official Catholic Teachings: Love and Sexuality* (McGraw, Wilmington, NC, 1978), pp. 99–100, and in *The Human Body: Papal Teachings*, selected by the monks of Solesmes (St Paul Editions, Boston, 1960).

54 Lesley Brown's worries are described in *A Matter of Life*, p. 160. The letter to Carl Wood is quoted from *Test-Tube Conception*, p. 30, and the comments by the Brennans from *In Vitro Fertilization: Problems and Possibilities*, pp. 12 and 16.

56 The words of Pius XII are taken from an address given on 29 April 1949. This and the passage from the 1975 Vatican Declaration on Certain Questions Concerning Sexual Ethics are quoted by Laurence Fitzgerald, 'Test Tube Morality in the Final Analysis'. For the theologians mentioned, see William Daniel, SJ, 'Sexual Ethics in Relation to IVF and ET', in Walters and Singer (eds.), *Test-Tube Babies*, p. 76; and Charles Curran, STD, in the *Appendix* to the HEW report, section 4, p. 8.

60 Margaret Tighe's comments were made in an interview with the authors, 29 November 1982.

61 The suggestion about cancer research was made by Roger Short; see the *Appendix* to the HEW report, section 10, p. 5. Leon Kass's arguments about cost are in the same *Appendix*, section 2, pp. 25–6.

63 For the claim that infertility is not a disease, see Leon Kass, 'Babies by Means of In Vitro Fertilization: Unethical Experiments on the Unborn?', *New England Journal of Medicine*, 285 (1971), p. 1177. Jan Brennan's contrary opinion is quoted in the article by Peter Roberts in *Test-Tube Babies*, p. 15.

65 The costs of renal dialysis are given by Priscilla Kincaid-Smith, 'Commentary on Session 2: Allocation of Health Care Resources' in *In Vitro Fertilization: Problems and Possibilities*, p. 27. The costs of other procedures are taken from *Medical Benefits Schedule Book* (Australian Government Publishing Service, Canberra, 1982).

66 On the anxiety and depression caused by infertility, see Ada Armstrong, 'The Needs of Infertile People and the Place of a Self-

Help Initiative in Western Australia' and Jan Aitkin, 'Counselling Services for The Infertile', both in Patricia Harper and Jan Aitken (eds.), *A Child Is Not the 'Cure' For Infertility* (Institute of Family Studies, Melbourne, 1982). See also George Christie, 'Childlessness: psychological and social implications' in *Proceedings of the Second Australian Conference on Adoption* (Committee of the Second Australian Conference on Adoption, Melbourne, 1979), pp. 81–6. Isabel Bainbridge's comments come from 'With Child in Mind', *Test-Tube Babies*, pp. 123–4; Barbara Menning's are from Helen Holmes, Betty Hoskins, and Michael Gross (eds.), *The Custom-Made Child?* (Humana Press, Clifton, NJ, 1981), p. 263.

3　IVF: Beyond the simple case

70　See Gillian Hanscombe, 'The Right to Lesbian Parenthood', *Journal of Medical Ethics*, ix (1983), 3, pp. 133–5.

72　On the extent of AID see Russell Scott, *The Body as Property* (Allen Lane, London, 1981), p. 199; John Leeton, 'The development and Demand for AID in Australia', in C. Wood (ed.), *Artificial Insemination By Donor* (no publisher, place, or date given), p. 11.

73　The risk of unwitting incest is discussed by Scott in *The Body as Property*, p. 210, and by David Danks, 'Genetic Considerations', in C. Wood (ed.), *Artificial Insemination By Donor*, pp. 101–2. On the problem of secrecy, see R. Snowden and G. D. Mitchell, *The Artificial Family* (Allen and Unwin, London, 1981), pp. 82–5, and Alison McMichael, 'Social Aspects' in *Artificial Insemination By Donor*, pp. 81–93.

74　Robyn Rowland, 'Attitudes and Opinions of Donors on an Artificial Insemination by Donor (AID) Programme' (unpublished typescript).

77　The pregnancy from a donor egg was reported in Alan Trounson and others, 'Pregnancy established in an infertile patient after transfer of a donated embryo fertilised in vitro', *British Medical Journal*, 286 (1983), pp. 835–8. Since donor sperm was used, the case was both a donated egg and a donated embryo. The subsequent correspondence appeared in the same volume of the *British Medical Journal*, pp. 1351–2.

78–9　For details of the opinion polls, see the notes to Ch. 1, pp. 32–4. The first successful intra-uterine transfers were reported in J. Buster *et al.*, 'Non-surgical transfer of in vivo fertilized donated ova to five infertile women: report of two pregnancies', *The Lancet*, July 1983, ii, pp. 223–4.

80　The debate over blood donation was stimulated by Richard Titmuss's key book, *The Gift Relationship* (Allen & Unwin, London, 1970). The suggestion that a voluntary system may use up the 'scarce resources' of altruism was made by Kenneth Arrow, 'Gifts and Exchanges', *Philosophy and Public Affairs*, 1 (1972) and criticized by Peter Singer, 'Altruism and Commerce', *Philosophy and Public Affairs*, 2 (1973). For a more recent assessment see Piet J. Hagen, *Blood: Gift or Merchandise* (Alan R. Liss, New York, 1982). Nozick's remark comes from his *Anarchy, State and Utopia* (Basic Books, New York, 1974), p. 163.

84 For the information on obtaining eggs from patients undergoing sterilization we are indebted to Dr Anne McLaren of the MRC Mammalian Development Unit, London.

86 On rate of cleavage and implantation, see Alan Trounson and others, 'Effect of delayed insemination on *in vitro* fertilization, culture and transfer of human embryos', *Journal of Reproduction and Fertility*, 64 (1982), pp. 285–94.

87 The argument beginning on this page was previously published in Helga Kuhse and Peter Singer, 'The Moral Status of the Embryo', in *Test-Tube Babies*, pp. 57–63.

97 On the development of the foetus to consciousness, see Clifford Grobstein, *From Chance to Purpose*, pp. 86–8. The expert opinion referred to is that of T. Humphrey, 'Function of The Nervous System During Pre-natal Life', in U. Stave (ed.), *Prenatal Physiology* (Plenum, New York, 1978), pp. 651–83.

99–100 Accounts of the method used by Wood's team to produce the first pregnancy from a frozen embryo were published in *The Age* (Melbourne), 3 May 1983. The subsequent miscarriage of the pregnancy was reported in *The Age*, 18 July 1983 and the *Canberra Times* of the same date. Edwards and Steptoe describe their earlier, unsuccessful efforts in *A Matter of Life*, pp. 153–4. A second pregnancy from a frozen embryo has been reported from Denmark (*Canberra Times*, 18 July 1983), and Wood's team has also announced another (*The Australian*, 22 October 1983).

101 On the risk of freezing leading to abnormal babies, see John Biggers, '*In Vitro* Fertilization, Embryo Culture and Embryo Transfer in the Human', HEW report, *Appendix*, section 8, pp. 34–5. The opinions of Alan Trounson and Robert Edwards were given in personal communications: for Grobstein's comment, see *New Scientist*, 7 October 1982.

102–3 For the statements of the NH & MRC and the BMA, see Appendix 1.

104 See Austin Asche, 'Legal Problems arising from AID, IVF and Related Procedures', in Frank Di Giantomasso (ed.), *Ethical Implica-*

tions in the Use of Donor Sperm, Eggs and Embryos in the Treatment of Human Infertility* (Monash Centre for Human Bioethics, Melbourne, 1983), pp. 57–66.

4 Surrogate motherhood

109 The case of Stefan and Nadia is taken from Noel Keane and Denis Breo, *The Surrogate Mother* (Everest House, New York, 1981). Other cases of surrogacy described in this chapter are taken from the same source, unless otherwise stated.

111 On the decision of the ethics committee of the Queen Victoria Medical Centre, see *The Age* (Melbourne), 25 April and 13 May 1981. For the guide-lines of the NH & MRC and BMA, see Appendix I.

116 The quotes are from pp. 15 and 24 of *The Surrogate Mother*.

117 The 'drug addict and lesbian' remark is on p. 107 of *The Surrogate Mother*, and the more favourable final assessment on p. 131.

119 Keane quotes the editorial on p. 265 of *The Surrogate Mother*. The Stiver–Malahoff case was reported in *The Herald* (Melbourne), 1 February 1983.

120–1 Keane's statement about unenforceable contracts is on p. 234. The British case was reported in *The Times* (London), 21 June 1978, and is briefly discussed by Douglas Cusine, ' "Womb-Leasing"; Some Legal Implications', *New Law Journal*, 24 August 1978, pp. 824–5.

124 The Crozel surrogate pregnancy was reported in *The Times* (London), 29 April 1983.

5 Ectogenesis

131 Details of the birth of Kim Bland were kindly supplied by Dr Victor Yu, Director of the Neonatal Intensive Care Unit at the Queen Victoria Medical Centre, and checked by Faye Bland.

132–3 Edwards's description of the embryo is from *A Matter of Life*, p. 131. For the claim that it would have developed further, see Robert Edwards, 'The Case for Studying Human Embryos and their Constituent Tissues *in vitro*', in Robert Edwards and Jean Purdy (eds.), *Human Conception In Vitro* (Academic Press, London, 1982), p. 379. Dennis New's work with rodent embryos was reported in *The Age* (Melbourne), 10 June 1983, citing a *Sunday Times* (London) report.

136–7 Shulamith Firestone's views are taken from *The Dialectic of Sex* (Bantam, New York, 1971). The passage quoted is from p. 206. See also pp. 8–12, 197–9.

139 For Edwards's suggestion, see his paper in *Human Conception in Vitro*, pp. 380–2.

143 Firestone's description of pregnancy is on pp. 198–9 of *The Dialectic of Sex*.

6 Cloning and sex selection

151 Rorvik does not give a source for the quotation from Lederberg and we have been unable to trace it. The cloning of cattle by embryo division has been carried out at Colorado State University, Fort Collins. See *The Herald* (Melbourne), 9 May 1983.

153 On the cloning of frogs, see Robert Gilmore McKinnell, *Cloning: A Biologist Reports* (University of Minnesota Press, Minneapolis, 1979), Ch. 3. On the inability to do this with cells from adult frogs, see p. 53. The initial report of successful cloning from a mouse embryo was in *Science*, 211 (1981), p. 375: for later doubts about some of Illmensee's work see *Neue Zürcher Zeitung* (Zurich), 28 May 1983.

154 On the heritability of intelligence, see, for example, Ned Block and Gerald Dworkin (eds.), *The IQ Controversy* (Pantheon, New York, 1976).

155 Edwards's proposal that we clone in order to type embryos was made in 'The Ethical, Scientific and Medical Implications of Human Conception In Vitro', an unpublished paper he read to the Pontifical Academy of Sciences, Vatican, 1982, p. 22. On determining the sex of the mouse embryo, see L. Singh and K. Jones, 'Sex Reversal in the Mouse', *Cell*, 28 (1982), pp. 205–16.

162–3 For the guide-lines referred to, see Appendix 1. The reference to them in the *Hastings Center Report* was in volume 13, no. 1 (February 1983), p. 2.

167 Aristotle's theory of sex determination is based on a complex account of bodily 'fluidity', with more fluid bodies leading to female offspring, and bodily fluidity itself being increased by southerly winds. See *Generation of Animals*, IV, ii, 767a (Loeb Classical Library, Heine-mann, London, 1953, tr. A. Peck), p. 397.

168 The experience of the genetics centre is described by Haig Kazazian, Jr in 'Prenatal Diagnosis for Sex Choice: A Medical View', *Hastings Center Report*, 10, 1 (1980), pp. 17–18.

169 Nakajima's work on sperm separation was reported in *The Age* (Melbourne), 12 May 1983. For an overview of current work on various methods of sex selection, see M. Ruth Nentwig, 'Technical Aspects of Sex Pre-selection' in Helen Holmes, Betty Hoskins, and Michael Gross (eds.), *The Custom-Made Child* (Humana Press, Clifton,

NJ, 1981), pp. 181–6. For examples of female infanticide among the Netsilik Eskimo, see Asen Balikci, *The Netsilik Eskimo* (Natural History Press, Garden City, NJ, 1970), pp. 148–9; and among the Japanese, Thomas C. Smith, *Nakahara: Family Farming and Population in a Japanese Village* (Stanford University Press, Stanford, 1977), Ch. 5.

Etzioni's discussion of sex selection is in 'Sex Control, Science and Society', *Science*, 161 (1968), pp. 1107–12 and reprinted in Amitai Etzioni, *Genetic Fix* (Harper & Row, New York, 1975), pp. 223–39. For a more concerned, feminist perspective see Roberta Steinbacher, 'Futuristic Implications of Sex Preselection', in *The Custom-Made Child*, pp. 187–91. Surveys on how parents would choose are criticized by Tabitha Powledge, 'Unnatural Selection: On Choosing Children's Sex', also in *The Custom-Made Child*. pp. 193–9.

170 Ehrlich's comment is from *The Population Bomb* (Ballantine, New York, revised edition, 1971), p. 133. See also J. Postgate, 'Bat's Chance in Hell', *New Scientist*, 58 (5 April 1973), pp. 12–13. For reports of the current practice of female infanticide in China, see 'Why Female Infanticide Still Exists in Socialist China', *Women of China*, (Peking) May 1983.

7 Genetic engineering

172 The opening quotation is from Nicholas Wade, *The Ultimate Experiment* (Walker, New York, 1977), p. 2.

174 The passage from *Frankenstein* is on p. 227 of the Everyman edition (J. M. Dent & Sons, London, 1912). Erwin Chargaff is quoted by Liebe Cavalieri, 'New Strains of Life—or Death', *New York Times*, 22 August 1976, Magazine section, pp. 8, 68; Robert Sinsheimer is quoted by Bernard Dixon, 'Tinkering with genes', *Spectator*, 235 (1975), p. 289. I owe both these references to *Splicing Life: A Report on the Social and Ethical Issues of Genetic Engineering with Human Beings*, issued by the President's Commission for the Study of Ethical Problems in Medicine and Biomedical and Behavioural Research, (US Govt Printing Office, Washington, DC, 1982), pp. 15, 62. The 1980 survey is also mentioned in *Splicing Life*, p. 71, referring to John Walsh, 'Public Attitude to Science is Yes, but—', *Science*, 215 (1982), p. 270.

175 *Splicing Life*, p. 2.

176 The 'gloved hands' metaphor comes from Francis Crick, 'Nucleic Acids' in D. Freifelder (ed.), *Recombinant DNA* (W. H. Freeman, San Francisco, 1978), p. 8. I owe the reference to Jeremy Cherfas, *Man Made Life* (Blackwell, Oxford, 1982), p. 16: this book is a useful

introduction to the background and current techniques of genetic engineering.

177 On the commercial production of genetically engineered human insulin, see *New York Times*, 30 October 1982.

179 See R. D. Palmiter and others, 'Dramatic growth of mice that developed from eggs micro-injected with metallothionein growth hormone fusion genes', *Nature*, 300 (1982), pp. 611–15.

180 The Letter from Three General Secretaries is published as an appendix to *Splicing Life*, on pp. 95–6. The Commission's summary of the evidence of the theologians is on pp. 53–4.

184 Jonathan Glover's lucid and stimulating book, *What Sort of People Should There Be?* (Penguin, Harmondsworth, 1984) was not available to us until after the text of this book had been completed. We find, however, that on several points Glover has reached conclusions similar to our own. Like us, he is doubtful about the sharpness of the distinction between improving humankind and eliminating faults—or as he puts it, the 'positive–negative distinction'. His example is different from ours, and worth citing. Suppose, he says, that a genetic disposition to depressive mental illness is found to be associated with the production of lower levels of an enzyme than are produced in normal people. To use genetic engineering to bring such a person's enzyme production into the normal range would then presumably be a case of 'negative' genetic engineering—eliminating a fault. But suppose that variations in the level of the enzyme in normal people correlated with ordinary differences in the tendency to be cheerful or to be depressed. 'Is it clear', Glover asks, 'that a sharp distinction can be drawn between raising someone's enzyme level so that it falls within the normal range and raising someone else's level from the bottom of the normal range to the top?' (p. 32). Nor does Glover think that, in so far as the distinction can be drawn, there is any objection of principle (as distinct from objections based on possible dangers) to changing human nature (pp. 55–6).

186 The free market approach to genetic engineering is suggested by Robert Nozick, *Anarchy, State and Utopia*, p. 315n. But even he, significantly, finds difficulties with a purely libertarian system.

189 Again, there are striking parallels between the conclusion we have reached favouring a mixed system, and the view reached independently by Jonathan Glover. His light-hearted summary of the options is worth quoting: 'Decision-taking by a central committee (perhaps of a dozen elderly men) can be thought of as a 'Russian' model. The genetic supermarket (perhaps with genotypes being sold by TV

commercials) can be thought of as an 'American' model. The mixed system may appeal to Western European social democrats' (p. 51n).

8 How do we handle these issues?

195 Burke's remarks, from his 'Speech to the Electors of Bristol, November 3, 1774' can be found in his *Works* (Bohn, London, 1883–90), I, pp. 446–7.

196 Of the inquiries referred to, the British Commission of Inquiry, chaired by the Oxford philosopher Mary Warnock, is the most extensive in scope and is not expected to report until 1985. The New South Wales committee is under the chairmanship of Russell Scott, a New South Wales Law Reform Commissioner and author of *The Body as Property* (Allen Lane, London, 1981). The Queensland committee is headed by a judge, Mr Justice Demack. At the time of writing it is not clear when these committees will report. All the other inquiries mentioned have reported (although the Victorian committee will issue further reports on issues other than those already covered) and their reports are included in full or in abridged form in Appendix 1.

196–7 See Ithiel de Sola Pool, 'The New Censorship of Social Research', *The Public Interest*, Spring 1980, pp. 57–66.

198 The passages quoted from the Board's report can be found in the extract in Appendix 1.

199 This section draws on some earlier writings by Peter Singer, especially 'Moral Experts', *Analysis*, 32 (1972), pp. 115–17 and 'Bioethics: The Case of the Fetus', *New York Review of Books*, 15 August 1976.

SELECT BIBLIOGRAPHY

This bibliography is intended as a guide for those who wish to read more widely on the ethical issues discussed in this book. Hence it includes only the more significant books and articles. There are several items referred to in the text which we have not considered sufficiently central to be listed here: full references to such items can be found in the Notes on Sources. Items of a purely scientific or technical nature have also been excluded.

In vitro fertilization

Books

Margaret Brumby (ed.), *Proceedings of the Conference: In Vitro Fertilization: Problems and Possibilities* (Monash Centre for Human Bioethics, Clayton, Victoria, 1982).

Thomas Carney, *Instant Evolution* (University of Notre Dame Press, Notre Dame, 1980).

Robert Edwards and Jean Purdy (eds.), *Human Conception in Vitro* (Academic Press, London, 1982).

Robert Edwards and Patrick Steptoe, *A Matter of Life* (Sphere, London, 1981).

R. H. Glass and R. J. Ericsson, *Getting Pregnant in the 1980s: New Advances in Infertility Treatment and Sex Preselection* (University of California Press, Berkeley, 1983).

Clifford Grobstein, *From Chance to Purpose: An Appraisal of External Human Fertilization* (Addison-Wesley, Reading, Mass., 1981).

Helen Holmes, Betty Hoskins, and Michael Gross (eds.), *The Custom-Made Child* (Humana Press, Clifton, NJ, 1981).

Ted Howard and Jeremy Rifkin, *Who Should Play God?* (Dell, New York, 1980).

William Walters and Peter Singer (eds.), *Test-Tube Babies* (Oxford University Press, Melbourne, 1982).

Carl Wood and Ann Westmore, *Test-Tube Conception* (Hill of Content, Melbourne, 1983).

Reports

Note: This list does not include brief reports which have been reprinted in full in Appendix 1 of this book.

Ethics Advisory Board, Department of Health, Education and Welfare, US Government, 'Protection of Human Subjects: HEW Support of Human In Vitro Fertilization and Embryo Transfer', *Federal Register*, 18 June 1979, 35033–35058. *Note*: The written submissions have been published separately as *Appendix: HEW Support of Research Involving Human In Vitro Fertilization and Embryo Transfer* (US Govt Printing Office, Washington, DC, 1979).

Victorian Government Committee to Consider the Social, Ethical and Legal Issues Arising from In Vitro Fertilization, *Interim Report*, published by the Committee, Melbourne, 1982.

Articles

Isabel Bainbridge, 'With Child in Mind: The experiences of a potential IVF mother', in William Walters and Peter Singer (eds.), *Test-Tube Babies* (Oxford University Press, Melbourne, 1982), pp. 119–27.

Jan and Len Brennan, 'Case Study: Becoming IVF Parents', in Margaret N. Brumby (ed.), *In Vitro Fertilization: Problems and Possibilities* (Monash Centre for Human Bioethics, Clayton, Victoria, 1982), pp. 12–16.

Margaret Brumby, 'Australian Community Attitudes to In Vitro Fertilization', *Medical Journal of Australia*, 2, no. 12 (1983), pp. 650–3.

The Catholic Bishops of Victoria, 'Submission to IVF Inquiry', *The Advocate* (Melbourne), 19 August 1982.

Charles Curran, 'In Vitro Fertilization and Embryo Transfer: From a Perspective of Moral Theology', in Ethics Advisory Board, *Appendix: HEW Support of Research Involving Human In Vitro Fertilization and Embryo Transfer*, (US Government Printing Office, Washington, DC, 1979), Ch. 4, 33 pp.

William Daniel, 'Sexual Ethics in relation to IVF and ET: The fitting use of human reproductive power', in Walters and Singer, op. cit., pp. 71–8.

R. G. Edwards, 'Fertilization of Human Eggs In Vitro: Morals, Ethics and the Law', *Quarterly Review of Biology*, 49 (1974), pp. 3–26.

R. G. Edwards, 'The Ethical, Scientific and Medical Implications of Human Conception In Vitro', unpublished paper read to the Pontifical Academy of Sciences, Vatican, 1982.

Fr. Laurence Fitzgerald, 'Test Tube Morality in the Final Analysis' *The Advocate* (Melbourne), 5 April 1982.

Gallup Poll, 'Public Opinion Survey', in Ethics Advisory Board, op. cit., Ch. 21, 4 pp.

Samuel Gorovitz, '*In Vitro* Fertilization: Sense and Nonsense', in Ethics Advisory Board, op. cit., Ch. 3, 30 pp.

Clifford Grobstein, 'Statement to the HEW Ethics Advisory Board', in Ethics Advisory Board, op. cit., Ch. 24, 6 pp.

Clifford Grobstein, Michael Flower, and John Mendeloff, 'External (In Vitro) Human Fertilization: A Five-Year Assessment of a New Reproductive Technology', unpublished typescript: a condensed version has been published as 'External Human Fertilization: An Evaluation of Policy', *Science*, 222 (14 October 1983), pp. 127–33.

John Harris, 'In Vitro Fertilization: The Ethical Issues I', *Philosophical Quarterly*, 33 (1983), pp. 217–37.

Louis Harris Associates, 'A Study of the Attitudes of American Women Toward the "Test-Tube" Procedure and Related Matters, Summary Section', in Ethics Advisory Board, op. cit., Ch. 22, 9 pp.

Stanley Hauerwas, 'Theological Reflections on In Vitro Fertilization', in Ethics Advisory Board, op. cit., Ch. 5, 20 pp.

John Henley, 'IVF and the Human Family: Possible and likely consequences', in Walters and Singer, op. cit., pp. 79–87.

Brian Johnstone, 'The Moral Status of the Embryo', in Walters and Singer, op. cit., pp. 49–56.

H. W. Jones, 'The Ethics of in-vitro Fertilization—1981' in R. G. Edwards and Jean Purdy (eds.), *Human Conception In Vitro* (Academic Press, London, 1982), pp. 351–7 (with discussion following, pp. 359–70).

Leon Kass, 'Babies by Means of In Vitro Fertilization: Unethical Experiments on the Unborn?', *New England Journal of Medicine*, 285 (1971), pp. 1174–9.

Leon Kass, 'Making Babies: The New Biology and the "Old" Morality', *The Public Interest*, 26 (1972), pp. 18–56.

Leon Kass, '"Making Babies" Revisited', *The Public Interest*, 54 (1979), pp. 32–60.

Leon Kass, 'Ethical Issues in Human *In Vitro* Fertilization, Embryo Culture and Research, and Embryo Transfer', in Ethics Advisory Board, op. cit., Ch. 2, 37 pp.

Helga Kuhse, 'An Ethical Approach to IVF & ET: What ethics is all about', in Walters and Singer, op. cit., pp. 22–35.

Helga Kuhse, 'The Ethics of In Vitro Fertilization', in Margaret Brumby, op. cit., pp. 54–61.

Helga Kuhse and Peter Singer, 'The Moral Status of the Embryo', in Walters and Singer, op. cit., pp. 49–63.

Sid Leiman, 'Human *In Vitro* Fertilization: A Jewish Perspective', in Ethics Advisory Board, op. cit., Ch. 6, 14 pp.

G. D. Mitchell, 'Comment', *Journal of Medical Ethics*, ix (1983), 4, pp. 196–8.

John Morgan, 'The Created Individual: Are basic notions of humanity threatened?', in Walters and Singer, op. cit., pp. 88–96.

Kay Oke and Jan Aitken, 'The Implications of IVF for the Individual', in Margaret Brumby, op. cit., pp. 67–71.

Paul Ramsey, 'Shall We "Reproduce"?', *Journal of the American Medical Association*, 220 (1972), pp. 1346–50 and 1480–5.

Paul Ramsey, 'Testimony on *In Vitro* Fertilization', in Ethics Advisory Board, op. cit., Ch. 7, 31 pp.

Alan Rassaby, 'In Vitro Fertilization: The New Technology, A Question of Inadequate Legal Protection for Child/Parent', in Margaret Brumby, op. cit., pp. 81–8.

J. N. Santamaria, 'In Vitro Fertilization and Embryo Transfer: A Perspective Based on Human Life and Human Rights', in Margaret Brumby, op. cit., pp. 48–53.

J. Schlesselman, 'How Does One Assess the Risk of Abnormalities from Human In Vitro Fertilization?', *American Journal of Obstetrics and Gynaecology*, 135 (1979), pp. 135–48, and also in Ethics Advisory Board, op. cit., Ch. 17, 63 pp.

Peter Singer and Deane Wells, '*In Vitro* Fertilization: The Major Issues', *Journal of Medical Ethics*, ix (1983), 4, pp. 192–9.

Alan Trounson, 'Current Perspectives and Future Prospects of *In Vitro* Fertilization', in Margaret Brumby, op. cit., pp. 41–7.

Alan Trounson, Carl Wood, and John Leeton, 'Freezing of Embryos: An Ethical Obligation', *Medical Journal of Australia*, 2 October 1982, pp. 332–3.

Le Roy Walters, 'Human In Vitro Fertilization: A Review of The Literature', *Hastings Center Report*, 9 (1979), No. 4, pp. 24–43.

Le Roy Walters, 'Ethical Issues in Human *In Vitro* Fertilization and Research involving Human Embryos', in Ethics Advisory Board, op. cit., Ch. 1, 52 + 14 pp.

William Walters and Peter Singer, 'Conclusions—and Costs', in Walters and Singer, op. cit., pp. 128–41.

Mary Warnock, 'In Vitro Fertilization: The Ethical Issues II', *Philosophical Quarterly*, 33 (1983), pp. 238–49.

Peter Williams and Gordon Stevens, 'What Now for Test Tube Babies?', *New Scientist*, 4 February 1982, pp. 312–16.

Carl Wood, 'IVF—Biology, Ethics and Administration.', in Margaret N. Brumby, op. cit., pp. 4–11.

Jillian Wood, 'Criteria For Selection of IVF Couples', in Margaret Brumby, op. cit., pp. 19–22.

Further developments: embryo freezing; use of donated sperm, eggs, or embryos; surrogate motherhood

Books

Frank Di Giantomasso (ed.), *Proceedings of the Conference: Ethical Implications in the Use of Donor Sperm, Eggs and Embryos in the Treatment of Human Infertility* (Monash Centre for Human Bioethics, Melbourne, 1983).

Noel Keane and Denis Breo, *The Surrogate Mother* (Everest House, New York, 1981).

Russell Scott, *The Body as Property* (Allen Lane, London, 1981).

R. Snowden and G. D. Mitchell, *The Artificial Family* (Allen and Unwin, London, 1981).

Carl Wood (ed.), *Artificial Insemination by Donor* (no publication details given; available from Dept. of Obstetrics and Gynaecology, Queen Victoria Medical Centre, Melbourne).

Report

Victorian Government Committee to Consider the Social, Ethical and Legal Issues Arising from In Vitro Fertilization, *Report on Donor Gametes in IVF* (August 1983), published by the Committee, Melbourne, 1983.

Articles

Austin Asche, 'Legal Problems arising from A.I.D., I.V.F. and Related Procedures', in Frank Di Giantomasso (ed.), *Proceedings of the Conference: Ethical Implications in the Use of Donor Sperm, Eggs and Embryos in the Treatment of Human Infertility* (Monash Centre for Human Bioethics, Melbourne, 1983), pp. 57–66.

Douglas Cusine, '"Womb-Leasing": Some Legal Implications', *New Law Journal*, 24 August 1978, pp. 824–5.

D. M. Danks, 'Genetic Aspects', in Carl Wood (ed.), *Artificial Insemination by Donor* (no publication details given), pp. 94–102.

E. A. Erikson, 'Contracts to Bear a Child', *California Law Review*, 66 (1978), pp. 611–22.

Gillian Hanscombe, 'The Right to Lesbian Parenthood', *Journal of Medical Ethics*, ix (1983), 3, pp. 133–5.

Herbert Krimmel, 'The Case Against Surrogate Parenting', *Hastings Center Report*, 13 (October 1983), No. 5, pp. 35–9.

Julienne Lauer, 'Implications of the Adoption Model for A.I.D., Donor Eggs and Surrogate Motherhood', in Frank Di Giantomasso, op. cit., pp. 37–9.

John Leeton, 'Medical Aspects of the Use of Donor Sperm, Eggs and Embryos in the Treatment of Human Infertility', in Frank Di Giantomasso, op. cit., pp. 11–16.

Eva Learner, 'The Social and Psychological Implications of Donor Sperm and Eggs', in Frank Di Giantomasso, op. cit., pp. 40–8.

Alison McMichael, 'Social Aspects', in Carl Wood, op. cit., pp. 81–93.

Alan Rassaby, 'Surrogate Motherhood: The position and problems of substitutes', in Walters and Singer, op. cit., pp. 97–109.

John Robertson, 'Surrogate Mothers: Not so Novel After all', *Hastings Center Report*, 13 (October 1983), No. 5, pp. 28–34.

R. V. Short, 'Scientific Prospects for the Use of Donor Sperm, Eggs and Embryos in the Treatment of Human Infertility', in Frank Di Giantomasso, op. cit., pp. 4–9.

Alan Trounson and others, 'Pregnancy established in an infertile patient after transfer of a donated embryo fertilised in vitro', *British Medical Journal*, 286 (1983), pp. 835–8.

Alan Trounson and Linda Mohr, 'Human Pregnancy Following Cryopreservation, Thawing and Transfer of an Eight-Cell Embryo', *Nature*, 305 (20–6 October 1983), p. 707.

William Walters, 'Ethical Aspects', in Carl Wood, op. cit., pp. 103–8.

William Winslade, 'Surrogate Mothers: private right or public wrong?', *Journal of Medical Ethics*, vii (1981), 3, pp. 153–4.

Ectogenesis, cloning, sex selection, and genetic engineering

Books

Jeremy Cherfas, *Man Made Life* (Blackwell, Oxford, 1982).

Amitai Etzioni, *Genetic Fix* (Harper and Row, New York, 1975).

Shulamith Firestone, *The Dialectic of Sex* (Bantam, New York, 1971).

Joseph Fletcher, *The Ethics of Genetic Control* (Doubleday, New York, 1974).

Jonathan Glover, *What Sort of People Should There Be?* (Penguin, Harmondsworth, 1984).

Robert Gilmore McKinnell, *Cloning: A Biologist Reports* (University of Minnesota Press, Minneapolis, 1978).

Paul Ramsey, *Fabricated Man: The Ethics of Genetic Control* (Yale University Press, New Haven, 1970).

Jeremy Rifkin, *Algeny* (Viking, New York, 1983).

David Rorvik, *In His Image: The Cloning of a Man* (J. P. Lippincott, New York, 1978).

Mary Shelley, *Frankenstein* (J. M. Dent and Sons, London, 1912).

Nicholas Wade, *The Ultimate Experiment* (Walker, New York, 1977).

Report

President's Commission for the Study of Ethical Problems in Medicine and Biomedical and Behavioral Research, *Splicing Life: A Report on the Social and Ethical Issues of Genetic Engineering with Human Beings* (US Government Printing Office, Washington, DC, 1982).

Articles

R. G. Edwards, 'The Case for Studying Human Embryos and their Constituent Tissues *in vitro*', in R. G. Edwards and Jean Purdy (eds.), *Human Conception In Vitro* (Academic Press, London, 1982), pp. 371–87.

R. G. Edwards, 'The Ethical, Scientific and Medical Implications of Human Conception In Vitro', unpublished paper read to the Pontifical Academy of Sciences, Vatican, 1982.

Amitai Etzioni, 'Sex Control, Science and Society', *Science*, 161 (1968), pp. 1107–12.

Joseph Fletcher, 'Ethical Aspects of Genetic Controls', *New England Journal of Medicine*, 285 (1971), pp. 776–83.

Haig Kazazian, Jr., 'Prenatal Diagnosis for Sex Choice', *Hastings Center Report*, 10 (1980), 1, pp. 17–18.

M. Ruth Nentwig, 'Technical Aspects of Sex Preselection', in Helen Holmes, Betty Hoskins, and Michael Gross (eds.), *The Custom-made Child* (Humana Press, Clifton, NJ, 1981), pp. 181–6.

Tabitha Powledge, 'Unnatural Selection: On Choosing Children's Sex', in Helen Holmes, Betty Hoskins, and Michael Gross, op. cit., pp. 193–9.

Roberta Steinbacher, 'Futuristic Implications of Sex Preselection', in Helen Holmes, Betty Hoskins, and Michael Gross, op. cit., pp. 187–91.

William Walters, 'Cloning, Ectogenesis and Hybrids: Things to Come?', in William Walters and Peter Singer, *Test-Tube Babies* (Oxford University Press, Melbourne, 1982), pp. 110–18.

INDEX